2. Baked salmon with lemon and dill

Ingredients:

• 4 salmon fillets (about 4•6 oz each)
• 2 tbsp olive oil
• 2 tbsp fresh lemon juice
• 2 tsp dried dill
• 1 tsp garlic powder
• 1/2 tsp salt
• 1/4 tsp black pepper

Instructions:

1. Preheat oven to 400°F.

2. In a small bowl, whisk together the olive oil, lemon juice, dill, garlic powder, salt, and pepper.

3. Place the salmon fillets in a baking dish and pour the lemon•dill mixture over the top, making sure to coat the fish evenly.

4. Bake for 12•15 minutes, or until the salmon is opaque and flakes easily with a fork.

5. Serve immediately, garnished with extra lemon wedges and fresh dill if desired.

Nutritional Information (per serving):
• Calories: 250
• Total Fat: 14g
• Saturated Fat: 2g
• Cholesterol: 80mg
• Sodium: 400mg
• Total Carbs: 0g
• Protein: 26g

This baked salmon dish is a great source of lean protein and healthy fats. The lemon and dill add tons of flavor without adding many calories. It's a great option for a low•calorie, high•protein meal that can be enjoyed as part of a weight loss program.

3. Turkey lettuce wraps

Ingredients:

• 1 lb ground turkey
• 1 tbsp olive oil
• 1 onion, diced
• 3 cloves garlic, minced
• 1 tbsp low•sodium soy sauce
• 1 tbsp rice vinegar
• 1 tsp sesame oil
• 1 tsp grated ginger
• 1/4 tsp red pepper flakes (optional)
• Salt and pepper to taste
• 12•16 large lettuce leaves (such as romaine or bibb)
• Toppings (optional): shredded carrots, sliced cucumber, chopped green onions, toasted sesame seeds

Instructions:

1. In a large skillet, heat the olive oil over medium•high heat. Add the ground turkey and cook, breaking it up with a wooden spoon, until browned and cooked through, about 5•7 minutes.

2. Add the onion and garlic to the skillet and cook for 2•3 minutes, until the onion is translucent.

3. Stir in the soy sauce, rice vinegar, sesame oil, ginger, and red pepper flakes (if using). Season with salt and pepper to taste.

4. To serve, place a few spoonfuls of the turkey mixture into the center of a lettuce leaf. Top with desired toppings. Fold the lettuce leaf around the filling and enjoy.

Nutritional Information (per serving, without toppings):
• Calories: 150
• Total Fat: 7g
• Saturated Fat: 2g
• Cholesterol: 60mg
• Sodium: 300mg
• Total Carbs: 3g
• Protein: 20g

These turkey lettuce wraps are a great low•carb, high•protein option for a healthy meal. The lean ground turkey and fresh lettuce leaves make it a perfect choice for a weight loss•friendly dish.

Welcome to the ***0-Point Weight Loss Cookbook: Fresh, Flavorful, and Filling Recipes for Weight Loss Success.*** If you've ever struggled with dieting, felt deprived, or worried about counting every single calorie, you're not alone. This cookbook is here to change that narrative and make your weight loss journey enjoyable and sustainable.

In this book, you'll discover over 100 delicious recipes that are all zero points, designed to help you lose weight without feeling hungry or deprived. These recipes are not only healthy but also packed with flavor, ensuring that every meal is a delightful experience. Our goal is to provide you with a variety of dishes that are easy to prepare, nutritionally balanced, and satisfying to your taste buds.

The concept of zero-point foods comes from the idea that certain foods are so low in calories and high in nutrients that they can be consumed freely without impacting your weight loss efforts. By focusing on these foods, you can create meals that keep you full and energized throughout the day.

Why Zero-Point Recipes?

Zero-point recipes are a game-changer for anyone looking to lose weight effectively. Here's why:

- **1. *Simplicity:*** Forget about complex calculations and tedious tracking. With zero-point foods, you can enjoy generous portions without the hassle.

- **2. *Nutrient-Dense:*** These recipes are packed with essential vitamins, minerals, and fiber, ensuring you get the nutrition you need while shedding pounds.

- **3. *Satisfaction:*** Eating zero-point foods means you can fill your plate and enjoy hearty meals that leave you feeling satisfied and happy.

- **4. *Variety:*** With over 100 recipes, you'll never get bored. From breakfast to dinner, snacks to desserts, there's something for every taste and occasion.

Embarking on a weight loss journey doesn't mean you have to give up the joy of eating. With the 0-Point Weight Loss Cookbook, you can embrace a healthier lifestyle without sacrificing flavor or satisfaction. These recipes are designed to be more than just meals; they're a way to nourish your body, delight your senses, and achieve your weight loss goals.

So, get ready to explore a world of zero-point possibilities. Whether you're a seasoned cook or a kitchen novice, you'll find recipes that are easy to follow and rewarding to eat. Here's to your success and enjoyment on this journey to a healthier, happier you!

1. Grilled chicken breast with herbs

Ingredients:

• 4 boneless, skinless chicken breasts
• 2 tbsp olive oil
• 2 tsp dried oregano
• 2 tsp dried basil
• 1 tsp garlic powder
• 1 tsp salt
• 1/2 tsp black pepper

Instructions:

1. Preheat grill to medium•high heat.

2. In a small bowl, mix together the olive oil, oregano, basil, garlic powder, salt, and pepper.

3. Rub the seasoning mixture all over the chicken breasts, coating them evenly.

4. Grill the chicken for 5•7 minutes per side, or until cooked through and no longer pink in the center.

5. Let the chicken rest for 5 minutes before serving.

Nutritional Information (per serving):
• Calories: 200
• Total Fat: 8g
• Saturated Fat: 2g
• Cholesterol: 90mg
• Sodium: 450mg
• Total Carbs: 0g
• Protein: 30g

This grilled chicken dish is a great lean protein option that is low in calories and carbs, making it a 0 point meal for weight loss programs. The herbs and spices add lots of flavor without adding extra calories.

4. Vegetable stir•fry with tofu

Ingredients:

- 1 block (14 oz) extra•firm tofu, cubed
- 2 tbsp low•sodium soy sauce
- 1 tbsp rice vinegar
- 1 tsp sesame oil
- 1 tbsp olive oil
- 1 red bell pepper, sliced
- 1 cup broccoli florets
- 1 cup sliced mushrooms
- 1 cup snow peas or snap peas
- 3 cloves garlic, minced
- 1 tbsp grated ginger
- 2 tsp cornstarch
- 1/4 cup low•sodium vegetable broth
- Salt and pepper to taste
- Chopped green onions and sesame seeds for garnish (optional)

Instructions:

1. In a small bowl, combine the tofu, soy sauce, rice vinegar, and sesame oil. Toss to coat and set aside.

2. Heat the olive oil in a large skillet or wok over high heat. Add the bell pepper, broccoli, mushrooms, and snow peas. Stir•fry for 3•4 minutes until vegetables are crisp•tender.

3. Add the garlic and ginger and cook for 1 minute, until fragrant.

4. In a small bowl, whisk together the cornstarch and vegetable broth. Pour the mixture into the skillet and stir to coat the vegetables.

5. Add the marinated tofu and continue to cook for 2•3 minutes, until the sauce has thickened.

6. Season with salt and pepper to taste. Serve immediately, garnished with chopped green onions and sesame seeds if desired.

Nutritional Information (per serving):
- Calories: 180
- Total Fat: 9g
- Saturated Fat: 1g
- Cholesterol: 0mg
- Sodium: 350mg
- Total Carbs: 12g
- Protein: 15g

This vegetable stir•fry with tofu is a 0 point meal for weight loss programs. It's packed with fiber, protein, and nutrients from the vegetables and tofu, making it a healthy and satisfying option.

5. Zucchini noodles with marinara sauce

Ingredients:

• 4 medium zucchinis, spiralized or julienned into noodles
• 1 tbsp olive oil
• 3 cloves garlic, minced
• 1 (28 oz) can crushed tomatoes
• 2 tbsp tomato paste
• 1 tsp dried oregano
• 1/2 tsp dried basil
• 1/4 tsp red pepper flakes (optional)
• Salt and pepper to taste
• Grated Parmesan cheese for serving (optional)

Instructions:

1. In a large skillet, heat the olive oil over medium heat. Add the garlic and cook for 1 minute, until fragrant.

2. Add the spiralized or julienned zucchini noodles to the skillet. Cook for 3•5 minutes, stirring occasionally, until the noodles are tender but still have a bit of bite.

3. In a separate saucepan, combine the crushed tomatoes, tomato paste, oregano, basil, and red pepper flakes (if using). Season with salt and pepper to taste.

4. Bring the marinara sauce to a simmer and cook for 5•10 minutes, stirring occasionally, until thickened.

5. Divide the zucchini noodles among plates or bowls. Top with the warm marinara sauce. Serve immediately, garnished with grated Parmesan cheese if desired.

Nutritional Information (per serving, without Parmesan):
• Calories: 120
• Total Fat: 5g
• Saturated Fat: 1g
• Cholesterol: 0mg
• Sodium: 350mg
• Total Carbs: 12g
• Fiber: 3g
• Protein: 4g

This zucchini noodle dish is a 0 point meal for weight loss programs. The zucchini noodles are a low•calorie, low•carb alternative to traditional pasta, and the homemade marinara sauce is packed with flavor without added sugars or unhealthy fats.

6. Cauliflower rice stir•fry

Ingredients:

• 1 head of cauliflower, riced (about 4 cups riced cauliflower)
• 1 tbsp olive oil
• 1 onion, diced
• 3 cloves garlic, minced
• 1 cup diced bell pepper (any color)
• 1 cup sliced mushrooms
• 1 cup snow peas or snap peas
• 2 tbsp low•sodium soy sauce
• 1 tsp sesame oil
• 1/4 tsp red pepper flakes (optional)
• Salt and pepper to taste
• Chopped green onions and toasted sesame seeds for garnish (optional)

Instructions:

1. In a large skillet or wok, heat the olive oil over medium•high heat.

2. Add the riced cauliflower, onion, and garlic. Stir•fry for 3•4 minutes until the cauliflower is starting to soften.

3. Add the bell pepper, mushrooms, and snow peas. Continue to stir•fry for 3•5 minutes, until the vegetables are tender•crisp.

4. Stir in the soy sauce, sesame oil, and red pepper flakes (if using). Season with salt and pepper to taste.

5. Cook for 1•2 minutes more, until everything is heated through. Serve the cauliflower rice stir•fry immediately, garnished with chopped green onions and toasted sesame seeds if desired.

Nutritional Information (per serving):
• Calories: 100
• Total Fat: 5g
• Saturated Fat: 1g
• Cholesterol: 0mg
• Sodium: 300mg
• Total Carbs: 10g
• Fiber: 3g
• Protein: 4g

7. Egg white omelette with spinach and tomatoes

Ingredients:

- 6 egg whites
- 1 tsp olive oil
- 1 cup fresh spinach, chopped
- 1/2 cup cherry tomatoes, halved
- 2 tbsp crumbled feta cheese (optional)
- Salt and pepper to taste

Instructions:

1. In a small bowl, whisk the egg whites until frothy.

2. Heat the olive oil in a non•stick skillet over medium heat.

3. Pour the egg whites into the skillet and let them cook for 2•3 minutes, until the bottom is set.

4. Sprinkle the chopped spinach and halved cherry tomatoes over the top of the egg whites.

5. Use a spatula to gently fold the omelette in half.

6. Cook for an additional 2•3 minutes, until the omelette is cooked through.

7. Slide the omelette onto a plate and top with the crumbled feta cheese, if using.

8. Season with salt and pepper to taste.

Nutritional Information (per serving):
- Calories: 150
- Total Fat: 6g
- Saturated Fat: 2g
- Cholesterol: 0mg
- Sodium: 350mg
- Total Carbs: 5g
- Protein: 20g

This egg white omelette is a great option for a healthy, high•protein breakfast or brunch. The spinach and tomatoes add vitamins, minerals, and fiber, while the feta cheese provides a creamy, tangy flavor. It's a delicious and nutritious meal that can be enjoyed as part of a weight loss program.

8. Shrimp ceviche

Ingredients:

• 1 lb raw shrimp, peeled, deveined, and chopped
• 1 cup fresh lime juice (about 6•8 limes)
• 1/2 cup fresh orange juice
• 1 jalapeño, seeded and finely chopped
• 1 red onion, finely chopped
• 1 cup chopped tomatoes
• 1/2 cup chopped cilantro
• 1 avocado, diced
• Salt and pepper to taste

Instructions:

1. In a large non•reactive bowl (glass or stainless steel), combine the chopped shrimp, lime juice, and orange juice. Cover and refrigerate for 30•60 minutes, stirring occasionally, until the shrimp is opaque and "cooked" through the acid in the citrus juices.

2. Drain any excess liquid from the shrimp mixture.

3. Add the jalapeño, red onion, tomatoes, cilantro, and avocado. Gently toss to combine.

4. Season with salt and pepper to taste.

5. Serve chilled, with lettuce leaves or tortilla chips on the side (optional).

Nutritional Information (per serving):
• Calories: 150
• Total Fat: 6g
• Saturated Fat: 1g
• Cholesterol: 170mg
• Sodium: 300mg
• Total Carbs: 8g
• Fiber: 3g
• Protein: 18g

This shrimp ceviche is a 0 point meal for weight loss programs. It's a refreshing, flavorful dish that's packed with lean protein from the shrimp and healthy fats from the avocado. The citrus, vegetables, and herbs provide a boost of vitamins, minerals, and antioxidants.

9. Greek salad with grilled chicken

Ingredients:

- 4 boneless, skinless chicken breasts
- 1 tbsp olive oil
- 1 tsp dried oregano
- Salt and pepper to taste
- 6 cups chopped romaine lettuce
- 1 cup cherry tomatoes, halved
- 1/2 cup sliced cucumber
- 1/4 cup sliced red onion
- 1/4 cup pitted kalamata olives
- 2 tbsp crumbled feta cheese
- 2 tbsp lemon juice
- 1 tbsp red wine vinegar
- 1 tsp Dijon mustard
- 1 tsp dried oregano
- 2 tbsp olive oil

Instructions:

1. Preheat grill or grill pan to medium•high heat.

2. Rub the chicken breasts with 1 tbsp olive oil, 1 tsp dried oregano, and season with salt and pepper.

3. Grill the chicken for 5•7 minutes per side, or until cooked through. Let rest for 5 minutes, then slice or chop the chicken.

4. In a large salad bowl, combine the chopped romaine, cherry tomatoes, cucumber, red onion, and kalamata olives.

5. In a small bowl, whisk together the lemon juice, red wine vinegar, Dijon mustard, 1 tsp dried oregano, and 2 tbsp olive oil. Season with salt and pepper.

6. Drizzle the dressing over the salad and toss to coat. Top the salad with the grilled chicken and crumbled feta cheese.

Nutritional Information (per serving):
- Calories: 300
- Total Fat: 15g
- Saturated Fat: 3g
- Cholesterol: 90mg
- Sodium: 550mg
- Total Carbs: 10g
- Fiber: 3g
- Protein: 35g

This Greek salad with grilled chicken is a 0 point meal for weight loss programs. The combination of lean protein from the chicken, healthy fats from the olive oil and feta, and fiber•rich vegetables makes it a nutritious and satisfying option.

10. Cottage cheese with fresh berries

Ingredients:

• 1 cup low•fat or non•fat cottage cheese
• 1 cup mixed fresh berries (such as strawberries, blueberries, raspberries)
• 1 tsp honey (optional)

Instructions:

1. Scoop the cottage cheese into a bowl or serving dish.

2. Top the cottage cheese with the mixed fresh berries.

3. Drizzle the honey over the top, if using.

Nutritional Information (per serving):
• Calories: 180
• Total Fat: 4g
• Saturated Fat: 2g
• Cholesterol: 20mg
• Sodium: 360mg
• Total Carbs: 15g
• Fiber: 3g
• Protein: 20g

This cottage cheese and fresh berry dish is a 0 point meal for weight loss programs. It's a simple, nutrient•dense snack or light meal that provides a balance of protein, carbohydrates, and healthy fats.

The cottage cheese is a great source of lean protein, while the fresh berries are packed with fiber, vitamins, and antioxidants. The optional honey adds a touch of sweetness, but the dish is delicious without it as well.

This is a versatile and satisfying option that can be enjoyed as a breakfast, snack, or dessert. It's a great way to satisfy your sweet tooth while staying on track with your weight loss goals.

11. Steamed shrimp with cocktail sauce

Ingredients:

- 1 lb raw shrimp, peeled and deveined
- 1/2 cup low•sodium cocktail sauce
- 1 tbsp lemon juice
- 1 tsp prepared horseradish (optional)
- Salt and pepper to taste

Instructions:

1. Fill a large pot with 1•2 inches of water and bring to a boil over high heat.

2. Place the shrimp in a steamer basket or colander that fits inside the pot. Lower the steamer into the pot, making sure it doesn't touch the water.

3. Cover the pot and steam the shrimp for 3•5 minutes, until they are opaque and cooked through.

4. Remove the steamed shrimp from the pot and transfer to a serving platter.

5. In a small bowl, mix together the cocktail sauce, lemon juice, and horseradish (if using). Season with salt and pepper to taste.

6. Serve the steamed shrimp immediately, with the cocktail sauce on the side for dipping.

Nutritional Information (per serving):
- Calories: 120
- Total Fat: 1g
- Saturated Fat: 0g
- Cholesterol: 170mg
- Sodium: 450mg
- Total Carbs: 5g
- Protein: 22g

This steamed shrimp with cocktail sauce is a 0 point meal for weight loss programs. The shrimp is a lean, low•calorie protein source, and the cocktail sauce provides a flavorful dipping sauce without adding many calories. It's a simple, healthy, and satisfying option for a light meal or appetizer.

12. Grilled portobello mushrooms

Ingredients:

• 4 large portobello mushroom caps, stems removed
• 2 tbsp olive oil
• 2 tbsp balsamic vinegar
• 2 cloves garlic, minced
• 1 tsp dried thyme
• Salt and pepper to taste

Instructions:

1. Preheat grill or grill pan to medium•high heat.

2. In a shallow dish, whisk together the olive oil, balsamic vinegar, garlic, and thyme.

3. Add the portobello mushroom caps to the dish and turn to coat both sides in the marinade.

4. Grill the mushrooms for 4•5 minutes per side, or until they are tender and have grill marks.

5. Transfer the grilled portobello mushrooms to a plate and season with salt and pepper to taste.

6. Serve the grilled portobello mushrooms warm, as a main dish or side.

Nutritional Information (per serving):
• Calories: 80
• Total Fat: 5g
• Saturated Fat: 1g
• Cholesterol: 0mg
• Sodium: 15mg
• Total Carbs: 7g
• Fiber: 2g
• Protein: 3g

These grilled portobello mushrooms are a 0 point meal for weight loss programs. Portobello mushrooms are a great low•calorie, low•carb alternative to meat, and the simple marinade adds tons of flavor without adding many calories. Enjoy these grilled mushrooms as a main dish or a side to your favorite lean protein.

13. Baked cod with garlic and herbs

Ingredients:

- 4 cod fillets (about 6 oz each)
- 2 tbsp olive oil
- 3 cloves garlic, minced
- 2 tsp dried parsley
- 1 tsp dried thyme
- 1 tsp dried oregano
- 1/4 tsp red pepper flakes (optional)
- Salt and pepper to taste
- Lemon wedges for serving

Instructions:

1. Preheat oven to 400°F.

2. In a small bowl, mix together the olive oil, garlic, parsley, thyme, oregano, and red pepper flakes (if using).

3. Place the cod fillets in a baking dish and season with salt and pepper.

4. Spoon the garlic•herb oil mixture over the top of the cod, making sure to evenly coat the fillets.

5. Bake for 12•15 minutes, or until the cod is opaque and flakes easily with a fork.

6. Serve the baked cod immediately, with lemon wedges on the side.

Nutritional Information (per serving):
- Calories: 200
- Total Fat: 8g
- Saturated Fat: 1g
- Cholesterol: 80mg
- Sodium: 300mg
- Total Carbs: 0g
- Protein: 28g

This baked cod with garlic and herbs is a delicious and healthy option for a main dish. Cod is a lean, mild•flavored fish that is high in protein and low in calories. The simple garlic•herb topping adds tons of flavor without adding many calories or unhealthy fats. Serve this baked cod with a side of roasted vegetables or a fresh salad for a complete, well•balanced meal.

14. Turkey chili (using lean ground turkey)

Ingredients:

- 1 lb lean ground turkey
- 1 onion, diced
- 3 cloves garlic, minced
- 2 tbsp chili powder
- 1 tsp ground cumin
- 1 tsp dried oregano
- 1/2 tsp smoked paprika
- 1/4 tsp cayenne pepper (optional)
- 1 (15 oz) can diced tomatoes
- 1 (15 oz) can kidney beans, rinsed and drained
- 1 (15 oz) can black beans, rinsed and drained
- 1 cup low•sodium chicken or vegetable broth
- Salt and pepper to taste
- Chopped fresh cilantro for garnish (optional)

Instructions:

1. In a large pot or Dutch oven, cook the ground turkey over medium•high heat, breaking it up with a wooden spoon, until browned and cooked through, about 5•7 minutes.

2. Add the diced onion and minced garlic to the pot. Cook for 2•3 minutes, until the onion is translucent.

3. Stir in the chili powder, cumin, oregano, smoked paprika, and cayenne (if using). Cook for 1 minute to toast the spices.

4. Pour in the diced tomatoes, kidney beans, black beans, and chicken/vegetable broth. Stir to combine.

5. Bring the chili to a simmer and let it cook for 15•20 minutes, stirring occasionally, until thickened.

6. Season with salt and pepper to taste. Serve the turkey chili hot, garnished with chopped fresh cilantro if desired.

Nutritional Information (per serving):
- Calories: 250
- Total Fat: 5g
- Saturated Fat: 1g
- Cholesterol: 55mg
- Sodium: 550mg
- Total Carbs: 25g
- Fiber: 8g
- Protein: 25g

This turkey chili is a 0 point meal for weight loss programs. The lean ground turkey, beans, and vegetables provide a filling, nutrient•dense meal that is low in calories and high in protein and fiber. It's a delicious and satisfying option for a healthy lunch or dinner.

15. Caprese salad with balsamic glaze

Ingredients:

- 8 oz fresh mozzarella cheese, sliced
- 2 large tomatoes, sliced
- 1/4 cup fresh basil leaves
- 2 tbsp balsamic vinegar
- 1 tsp honey
- 1 tbsp olive oil
- Salt and pepper to taste

Instructions:

1. Arrange the sliced mozzarella and tomatoes on a serving platter or plate. Scatter the fresh basil leaves over the top.

2. In a small saucepan, combine the balsamic vinegar and honey. Bring to a simmer over medium heat and cook for 3·5 minutes, stirring occasionally, until the mixture has reduced and thickened into a glaze.

3. Drizzle the balsamic glaze over the caprese salad.

4. Drizzle the olive oil over the top of the salad.

5. Season with salt and pepper to taste. Serve immediately.

Nutritional Information (per serving):
- Calories: 150
- Total Fat: 10g
- Saturated Fat: 5g
- Cholesterol: 25mg
- Sodium: 250mg
- Total Carbs: 8g
- Fiber: 1g
- Protein: 10g

This caprese salad with balsamic glaze is a 0 point meal for weight loss programs. The fresh mozzarella, tomatoes, and basil provide a delicious and nutritious base, while the balsamic glaze adds a sweet and tangy flavor without adding many calories. It's a light, refreshing, and satisfying option that can be enjoyed as a main dish or a side salad.

16. Roasted butternut squash soup

Ingredients:

• 1 medium butternut squash, peeled, seeded, and cubed (about 4 cups)
• 2 tbsp olive oil
• 1 onion, diced
• 3 cloves garlic, minced
• 4 cups low•sodium vegetable or chicken broth
• 1 tsp ground cumin
• 1/2 tsp ground cinnamon
• 1/4 tsp ground nutmeg
• Salt and pepper to taste
• Chopped fresh parsley or chives for garnish (optional)

Instructions:

1. Preheat oven to 400°F.

2. Toss the cubed butternut squash with 1 tbsp of the olive oil on a baking sheet. Roast for 20•25 minutes, until tender and lightly browned.

3. In a large pot or Dutch oven, heat the remaining 1 tbsp of olive oil over medium heat. Add the diced onion and cook for 5 minutes, until translucent.

4. Add the minced garlic and cook for 1 minute, until fragrant.

5. Pour in the vegetable or chicken broth and add the roasted butternut squash, cumin, cinnamon, and nutmeg. Stir to combine.

6. Bring the soup to a simmer and cook for 10•15 minutes, until the flavors have melded.

7. Using an immersion blender or regular blender, puree the soup until smooth.

8. Season with salt and pepper to taste. Serve the roasted butternut squash soup warm, garnished with chopped fresh parsley or chives if desired.

Nutritional Information (per serving):
• Calories: 150
• Total Fat: 5g
• Saturated Fat: 1g
• Cholesterol: 0mg
• Sodium: 300mg
• Total Carbs: 25g
• Fiber: 5g
• Protein: 3g

This roasted butternut squash soup is a delicious and nutritious option. Butternut squash is a great source of fiber, vitamins, and antioxidants, and the roasting process brings out its natural sweetness. Enjoy this soup as a starter or a light main course.

17. Cucumber and tomato salad

Ingredients:

• 2 medium cucumbers, sliced
• 2 cups cherry or grape tomatoes, halved
• 1/2 red onion, thinly sliced
• 2 tbsp olive oil
• 2 tbsp red wine vinegar
• 1 tbsp lemon juice
• 1 tsp dried oregano
• 1/4 tsp salt
• 1/4 tsp black pepper
• 2 tbsp chopped fresh basil (optional)

Instructions:

1. In a large bowl, combine the sliced cucumbers, halved tomatoes, and thinly sliced red onion.

2. In a small bowl, whisk together the olive oil, red wine vinegar, lemon juice, dried oregano, salt, and black pepper.

3. Pour the dressing over the cucumber and tomato mixture and toss gently to coat.

4. If desired, sprinkle the chopped fresh basil over the top of the salad.

5. Refrigerate for at least 30 minutes to allow the flavors to meld. Serve chilled or at room temperature.

Nutritional Information (per serving):
• Calories: 80
• Total Fat: 5g
• Saturated Fat: 1g
• Cholesterol: 0mg
• Sodium: 150mg
• Total Carbs: 8g
• Fiber: 2g
• Protein: 2g

This cucumber and tomato salad is a refreshing and healthy side dish or snack. The combination of crisp cucumbers, juicy tomatoes, and tangy dressing makes for a light and flavorful salad. It's a great option for a low•calorie, low•carb meal or snack that can be enjoyed as part of a weight loss program.

18. Baked tilapia with mango salsa

Ingredients:

For the Mango Salsa:
• 1 ripe mango, diced
• 1/2 red onion, finely chopped
• 1 jalapeño, seeded and finely chopped
• 1/4 cup chopped fresh cilantro
• 2 tbsp lime juice
• 1/4 tsp salt

For the Tilapia:
• 4 tilapia fillets (about 4•6 oz each)
• 1 tbsp olive oil
• 1 tsp chili powder
• 1/2 tsp garlic powder
• 1/4 tsp salt
• 1/4 tsp black pepper

Instructions:

1. Preheat oven to 400°F.
2. Make the mango salsa: In a medium bowl, combine the diced mango, red onion, jalapeño, cilantro, lime juice, and 1/4 tsp salt. Stir to mix well and set aside.
3. Place the tilapia fillets on a baking sheet lined with parchment paper or foil. Brush the fillets with the olive oil and sprinkle with the chili powder, garlic powder, salt, and pepper.
4. Bake the tilapia for 12•15 minutes, or until it flakes easily with a fork.
5. Serve the baked tilapia warm, topped with the mango salsa.

Nutritional Information (per serving):
• Calories: 200
• Total Fat: 6g
• Saturated Fat: 1g
• Cholesterol: 60mg
• Sodium: 350mg
• Total Carbs: 12g
• Fiber: 2g
• Protein: 25g

This baked tilapia with mango salsa is a 0 point meal for weight loss programs. Tilapia is a lean, mild•flavored fish that is high in protein and low in calories. The mango salsa adds a sweet and tangy flavor without adding many calories. This dish is a great source of lean protein, healthy fats, and fiber, making it a nutritious and satisfying option for a weight loss•friendly meal.

19. Stuffed bell peppers with ground turkey

Ingredients:

- 2 tbsp tomato paste
- 1 tsp dried oregano
- 1/2 tsp dried basil
- 1/4 tsp red pepper flakes (optional)
- Salt and pepper to taste
- Shredded mozzarella cheese (optional)

- 4 bell peppers (any color), halved lengthwise and seeds/membranes removed
- 1 lb lean ground turkey
- 1 onion, diced
- 3 cloves garlic, minced
- 1 cup cooked brown rice
- 1 (14.5 oz) can diced tomatoes

Instructions:

1. Preheat oven to 375°F.

2. In a large skillet over medium heat, cook the ground turkey, onion, and garlic until the turkey is browned and the onion is translucent, about 5•7 minutes. Drain any excess fat.

3. Stir in the cooked brown rice, diced tomatoes, tomato paste, oregano, basil, and red pepper flakes (if using). Season with salt and pepper.

4. Stuff the hollowed•out bell pepper halves with the turkey and rice mixture, packing it in tightly.

5. Place the stuffed bell peppers in a baking dish. Cover with foil. Bake for 25•30 minutes, until the peppers are tender.

6. Remove the foil and top the stuffed peppers with shredded mozzarella cheese, if desired. Bake for an additional 5 minutes, until the cheese is melted. Serve the stuffed bell peppers warm.

Nutritional Information (per serving):
- Calories: 250
- Total Fat: 8g
- Saturated Fat: 2g
- Cholesterol: 70mg
- Sodium: 400mg
- Total Carbs: 20g
- Fiber: 5g
- Protein: 25g

This stuffed bell pepper dish is a 0 point meal for weight loss programs. The lean ground turkey, brown rice, and vegetables provide a filling, nutrient•dense meal that is low in calories and high in protein and fiber. It's a delicious and satisfying option for a healthy lunch or dinner.

20. Watermelon and feta salad

Ingredients:

- 4 cups cubed seedless watermelon
- 1 cup crumbled feta cheese
- 1/4 cup thinly sliced red onion
- 2 tbsp chopped fresh mint
- 1 tbsp balsamic glaze
- 1 tbsp olive oil
- 1/4 tsp salt
- 1/4 tsp black pepper

Instructions:

1. In a large bowl, gently toss together the cubed watermelon, crumbled feta cheese, sliced red onion, and chopped fresh mint.

2. Drizzle the balsamic glaze and olive oil over the salad. Sprinkle with salt and pepper.

3. Toss the salad gently to coat everything in the dressing.

4. Serve immediately or refrigerate until ready to serve.

Nutritional Information (per serving):
- Calories: 120
- Total Fat: 6g
- Saturated Fat: 3g
- Cholesterol: 15mg
- Sodium: 300mg
- Total Carbs: 12g
- Fiber: 1g
- Protein: 4g

This watermelon and feta salad is a refreshing and flavorful 0 point meal for weight loss programs. The juicy watermelon, salty feta, and fresh mint create a delightful balance of sweet and savory. The balsamic glaze and olive oil add a touch of richness without many calories. This salad is a great option for a light and healthy side dish or snack.

21. Poached chicken breast with steamed broccoli

Ingredients:

- 4 boneless, skinless chicken breasts
- 4 cups low•sodium chicken broth
- 1 bay leaf
- 2 sprigs fresh thyme
- 1 lemon, cut in half
- 1 lb broccoli florets
- 1 tbsp lemon juice
- Salt and pepper to taste

Instructions:

1. In a large pot, combine the chicken broth, bay leaf, thyme, and the juice from half of the lemon. Bring the liquid to a gentle simmer over medium heat.

2. Add the chicken breasts to the simmering broth. Poach the chicken for 12•15 minutes, or until cooked through and no longer pink in the center.

3. Remove the chicken from the broth and set aside. Discard the bay leaf and thyme.

4. In a steamer basket or saucepan with a small amount of water, steam the broccoli florets for 5•7 minutes, until tender•crisp.

5. Transfer the steamed broccoli to a serving dish and drizzle with the remaining lemon juice. Slice or shred the poached chicken and arrange it on the plate with the broccoli. Season the chicken and broccoli with salt and pepper to taste.

Nutritional Information (per serving):
- Calories: 200
- Total Fat: 3g
- Saturated Fat: 1g
- Cholesterol: 70mg
- Sodium: 300mg
- Total Carbs: 8g
- Fiber: 3g
- Protein: 32g

This poached chicken breast with steamed broccoli is a 0 point meal for weight loss programs. The lean protein from the chicken and the fiber and nutrients from the broccoli make this a filling and nutritious option. The simple preparation allows the natural flavors of the ingredients to shine through.

22. Greek yogurt parfait with fruit

Ingredients:

• 2 cups plain Greek yogurt
• 2 cups mixed fresh berries (such as strawberries, blueberries, raspberries)
• 2 tbsp honey (optional)
• 1/4 cup granola (optional)

Instructions:

1. In a parfait glass or bowl, layer the Greek yogurt and mixed berries, starting and ending with the yogurt.

2. If using, drizzle the honey over the layers.

3. Top with the granola, if desired.

4. Serve immediately or refrigerate until ready to serve.

Nutritional Information (per serving):
• Calories: 200
• Total Fat: 5g
• Saturated Fat: 2g
• Cholesterol: 15mg
• Sodium: 80mg
• Total Carbs: 25g
• Fiber: 4g
• Protein: 18g

This Greek yogurt parfait with fruit is a 0 point meal for weight loss programs. The Greek yogurt provides a good source of protein, while the fresh berries add fiber, vitamins, and natural sweetness. The optional honey and granola can add a touch of crunch and extra flavor, but the parfait is delicious without them as well.

This parfait makes for a satisfying and nutritious breakfast, snack, or dessert that can be enjoyed as part of a healthy weight loss plan. It's easy to prepare and can be customized with your favorite fruits and toppings.

23. Spinach and mushroom stuffed chicken breast

Ingredients:

• 4 boneless, skinless chicken breasts
• 8 oz fresh spinach, chopped
• 8 oz sliced mushrooms
• 2 cloves garlic, minced
• 1/4 cup grated Parmesan cheese
• 1 tsp dried thyme
• Salt and pepper to taste

Instructions:
1. Preheat oven to 400°F.

2. In a large skillet over medium heat, sauté the mushrooms and garlic until the mushrooms are tender, about 5 minutes. Add the chopped spinach and cook until wilted, about 2•3 minutes. Remove from heat and let cool slightly.

3. In a medium bowl, mix the sautéed spinach and mushroom mixture with the Parmesan cheese and dried thyme. Season with salt and pepper.

4. Slice each chicken breast horizontally to create a pocket. Stuff each pocket with the spinach and mushroom filling, dividing it evenly.

5. Place the stuffed chicken breasts in a baking dish and bake for 25•30 minutes, until the chicken is cooked through and the internal temperature reaches 165°F. Serve the spinach and mushroom stuffed chicken breasts immediately.

Nutritional Information (per serving):
• Calories: 200
• Total Fat: 5g
• Saturated Fat: 2g
• Cholesterol: 90mg
• Sodium: 350mg
• Total Carbs: 5g
• Fiber: 2g
• Protein: 35g

This spinach and mushroom stuffed chicken breast is a 0 point meal for weight loss programs. The lean chicken breast is filled with a flavorful, nutrient•dense stuffing that adds moisture and flavor without many calories. It's a delicious and satisfying main dish that can be enjoyed as part of a healthy, balanced diet.

24. Grilled swordfish with citrus marinade

Ingredients:

• 4 swordfish steaks (about 6 oz each)
• 1/4 cup fresh orange juice
• 2 tbsp fresh lemon juice
• 1 tbsp olive oil
• 2 cloves garlic, minced
• 1 tsp dried oregano
• 1/4 tsp salt
• 1/4 tsp black pepper

Instructions:

1. In a shallow baking dish or resealable plastic bag, combine the orange juice, lemon juice, olive oil, garlic, oregano, salt, and pepper. Add the swordfish steaks and turn to coat them evenly in the marinade.

2. Cover the dish or seal the bag and refrigerate for 30 minutes to 1 hour, turning the fish occasionally.

3. Preheat grill or grill pan to medium•high heat. Remove the swordfish from the marinade and discard the marinade.

4. Grill the swordfish for 4•5 minutes per side, or until it flakes easily with a fork and reaches an internal temperature of 145°F. Serve the grilled swordfish immediately.

Nutritional Information (per serving):
• Calories: 200
• Total Fat: 6g
• Saturated Fat: 1g
• Cholesterol: 60mg
• Sodium: 300mg
• Total Carbs: 3g
• Protein: 32g

This grilled swordfish with citrus marinade is a 0 point meal for weight loss programs. Swordfish is a lean, high•protein fish that is low in calories and carbs. The bright, tangy marinade adds tons of flavor without adding many calories. This dish is a great source of omega•3 fatty acids and other essential nutrients, making it a healthy and satisfying option for a weight loss•friendly meal.

25. Lentil soup

Ingredients:

- 1 tbsp olive oil
- 1 onion, diced
- 3 carrots, peeled and diced
- 3 celery stalks, diced
- 3 cloves garlic, minced
- 1 cup dried brown or green lentils, rinsed
- 6 cups low•sodium vegetable or chicken broth

- 1 (14.5 oz) can diced tomatoes
- 1 tsp dried thyme
- 1 tsp dried oregano
- 1/2 tsp smoked paprika
- Salt and pepper to taste
- Chopped fresh parsley for garnish (optional)

Instructions:

1. In a large pot or Dutch oven, heat the olive oil over medium heat. Add the diced onion, carrots, and celery. Cook for 5•7 minutes, until the vegetables are softened.

2. Add the minced garlic and cook for 1 minute, until fragrant.

3. Stir in the rinsed lentils, broth, diced tomatoes, thyme, oregano, and smoked paprika. Season with salt and pepper to taste.

4. Bring the soup to a boil, then reduce the heat and let it simmer for 20•25 minutes, or until the lentils are tender. Ladle the lentil soup into bowls and garnish with chopped fresh parsley, if desired.

Nutritional Information (per serving):
- Calories: 250
- Total Fat: 5g
- Saturated Fat: 1g
- Cholesterol: 0mg
- Sodium: 450mg
- Total Carbs: 35g
- Fiber: 12g
- Protein: 15g

This lentil soup is a 0 point meal for weight loss programs. Lentils are a great source of plant•based protein, fiber, and complex carbohydrates, making this soup a filling and nutritious option. The vegetables and spices add flavor and additional nutrients without many calories. Enjoy this hearty soup as a main dish or a side.

26. Quinoa salad with vegetables

Ingredients:

- 1 cup uncooked quinoa, rinsed
- 2 cups low•sodium vegetable or chicken broth
- 1 cup diced cucumber
- 1 cup cherry tomatoes, halved
- 1/2 cup diced red onion
- 1/2 cup diced bell pepper (any color)
- 1/4 cup chopped fresh parsley
- 2 tbsp olive oil
- 2 tbsp lemon juice
- 1 tsp Dijon mustard
- 1/2 tsp dried oregano
- Salt and pepper to taste

Instructions:

1. In a medium saucepan, combine the rinsed quinoa and broth. Bring to a boil, then reduce heat to low, cover, and simmer for 15•20 minutes, until the quinoa is tender and the liquid is absorbed.

2. Transfer the cooked quinoa to a large bowl and let it cool slightly.

3. Add the diced cucumber, cherry tomatoes, red onion, bell pepper, and chopped parsley to the bowl with the quinoa.

4. In a small bowl, whisk together the olive oil, lemon juice, Dijon mustard, and dried oregano. Season with salt and pepper.

5. Pour the dressing over the quinoa and vegetable mixture and toss gently to coat.

6. Serve the quinoa salad chilled or at room temperature.

This quinoa salad with vegetables is a 0 point meal for weight loss programs. Quinoa is a high•protein, high•fiber grain that provides complex carbohydrates, while the fresh vegetables add vitamins, minerals, and antioxidants. The simple lemon•Dijon dressing adds flavor without many calories. This salad is a great option for a light, nutrient•dense meal or side dish.

27. Tuna salad lettuce wraps

Ingredients:

- 2 (5 oz) cans of tuna, drained and flaked
- 2 tbsp plain Greek yogurt
- 1 tbsp Dijon mustard
- 1 tbsp lemon juice
- 2 tbsp finely chopped celery
- 2 tbsp finely chopped red onion
- 1 tbsp chopped fresh parsley
- Salt and pepper to taste
- 8·10 large lettuce leaves (such as romaine or bibb)

Instructions:

1. In a medium bowl, combine the flaked tuna, Greek yogurt, Dijon mustard, lemon juice, celery, red onion, and parsley. Mix well to combine.

2. Season the tuna salad with salt and pepper to taste.

3. Lay the lettuce leaves flat on a work surface. Scoop a portion of the tuna salad onto the center of each lettuce leaf.

4. Fold the sides of the lettuce leaf over the tuna salad and enjoy.

Nutritional Information (per serving, 2 lettuce wraps):
- Calories: 150
- Total Fat: 3g
- Saturated Fat: 1g
- Cholesterol: 35mg
- Sodium: 350mg
- Total Carbs: 5g
- Fiber: 2g
- Protein: 22g

These tuna salad lettuce wraps are a great 0 point meal for weight loss programs. The tuna provides lean protein, while the Greek yogurt and vegetables add flavor and nutrients without many calories. Serving the tuna salad in crisp lettuce leaves instead of bread or crackers keeps it low in carbs and calories. This is a satisfying and nutritious option for a light lunch or snack.

28. Broiled grapefruit with honey

Ingredients:

• 2 grapefruits, halved horizontally
• 2 tbsp honey
• 1/4 tsp ground cinnamon (optional)

Instructions:

1. Preheat your oven's broiler and position the oven rack about 6 inches from the heat source.

2. Cut the grapefruits in half horizontally and place them cut•side up on a baking sheet.

3. Drizzle 1 tsp of honey over the exposed flesh of each grapefruit half.

4. If desired, sprinkle a pinch of ground cinnamon over the honey.

5. Broil the grapefruit halves for 5•7 minutes, or until the honey is bubbly and starting to caramelize.

6. Carefully remove the baking sheet from the oven and let the grapefruit cool for a few minutes before serving.

Nutritional Information (per serving, 1/2 grapefruit):
• Calories: 80
• Total Fat: 0g
• Saturated Fat: 0g
• Cholesterol: 0mg
• Sodium: 0mg
• Total Carbs: 20g
• Fiber: 3g
• Protein: 1g

This broiled grapefruit with honey is a delicious and refreshing 0 point meal for weight loss programs. The natural sweetness of the grapefruit is enhanced by the caramelized honey, creating a simple yet satisfying dessert or snack. The cinnamon is optional, but it adds a warm, comforting flavor.

Grapefruits are a great source of vitamin C, fiber, and antioxidants, making this a nutritious and low•calorie option. Enjoy this broiled grapefruit as a healthy treat or a light addition to your weight loss meal plan.

29. Roasted Brussels sprouts with garlic

Ingredients:

• 1 lb Brussels sprouts, trimmed and halved
• 2 tbsp olive oil
• 3 cloves garlic, minced
• 1/2 tsp salt
• 1/4 tsp black pepper

Instructions:

1. Preheat your oven to 400°F.

2. In a large bowl, toss the trimmed and halved Brussels sprouts with the olive oil, minced garlic, salt, and black pepper until the sprouts are evenly coated.

3. Spread the Brussels sprouts in a single layer on a baking sheet.

4. Roast the Brussels sprouts for 20•25 minutes, tossing halfway, until they are tender and lightly browned.

5. Serve the roasted Brussels sprouts with garlic immediately.

Nutritional Information (per serving):
• Calories: 80
• Total Fat: 4g
• Saturated Fat: 1g
• Cholesterol: 0mg
• Sodium: 200mg
• Total Carbs: 8g
• Fiber: 3g
• Protein: 3g

These roasted Brussels sprouts with garlic are a 0 point meal for weight loss programs. Brussels sprouts are a nutrient•dense vegetable that is high in fiber, vitamins, and antioxidants. The simple preparation with olive oil, garlic, salt, and pepper allows the natural flavors of the Brussels sprouts to shine.

Roasting the Brussels sprouts brings out their natural sweetness and creates a delicious, crispy texture. This side dish is a great way to incorporate more vegetables into your diet while supporting your weight loss goals.

30. Apple slices with peanut butter

Ingredients:

• 1•2 apples, cored and sliced
• 2•3 tablespoons peanut butter

Instructions:

1. Wash and core the apples. Slice them into thin wedges or slices.

2. Spread a small amount of peanut butter onto each apple slice, about 1/2 to 1 teaspoon per slice.

3. Arrange the apple slices with peanut butter on a plate or platter.

That's it! This makes a quick, easy, and healthy snack. The crisp apple slices pair perfectly with the creamy peanut butter. You can use any type of apples you prefer. Some people also like to sprinkle a pinch of cinnamon over the top.

31. Edamame salad with sesame dressing

Ingredients:

- 2 cups shelled edamame, cooked and cooled
- 1 cup shredded carrots
- 1 cup thinly sliced cucumber
- 1/4 cup thinly sliced red onion
- 2 tablespoons chopped fresh cilantro
- 2 tablespoons rice vinegar
- 1 tablespoon sesame oil
- 1 tablespoon low•sodium soy sauce
- 1 teaspoon honey
- 1 teaspoon sesame seeds
- Salt and pepper to taste

Instructions:

1. In a large bowl, combine the cooked edamame, carrots, cucumber, red onion, and cilantro.

2. In a small bowl, whisk together the rice vinegar, sesame oil, soy sauce, and honey.

3. Pour the sesame dressing over the edamame salad and toss gently to coat.

4. Sprinkle the sesame seeds over the top.

5. Season with salt and pepper to taste.

6. Chill for at least 30 minutes before serving to allow the flavors to blend.

This edamame salad is refreshing, flavorful, and 0 points on most weight loss programs. The sesame dressing adds a nice nutty flavor without adding any extra points. Enjoy!

32. Cabbage soup

Ingredients:

- 1 head green cabbage, chopped
- 1 onion, diced
- 3 carrots, peeled and sliced
- 3 celery stalks, sliced
- 4 cups low•sodium vegetable or chicken broth
- 1 (14.5 oz) can diced tomatoes
- 2 cloves garlic, minced
- 1 tsp dried oregano
- 1 tsp dried basil
- Salt and pepper to taste

Instructions:

1. In a large pot or Dutch oven, sauté the onion, carrots, and celery in a small amount of broth or water over medium heat for 5•7 minutes until softened.

2. Add the chopped cabbage, garlic, oregano, and basil. Cook for 2•3 minutes, stirring frequently.

3. Pour in the vegetable or chicken broth and diced tomatoes. Bring the soup to a boil.

4. Reduce heat to low, cover and simmer for 20•25 minutes, until the cabbage is very tender.

5. Season with salt and pepper to taste.

This cabbage soup is packed with vegetables and fiber, yet very low in calories. It's a perfect 0 point soup for weight loss programs. You can enjoy a large bowl for very few points. Top with a sprinkle of Parmesan cheese if desired. Enjoy!

33. Baked apples with cinnamon

Ingredients:

• 4 medium apples, cored (leave bottom intact)
• 1/4 cup water
• 1 tsp ground cinnamon
• 1/4 tsp ground nutmeg (optional)
• 1 tbsp honey or maple syrup (optional)

Instructions:

1. Preheat oven to 375°F.

2. Core the apples, leaving the bottom intact so they can stand up. Place the cored apples in a baking dish.

3. In a small bowl, mix together the water, cinnamon, and nutmeg (if using).

4. Pour the cinnamon•water mixture into the baking dish, around the apples.

5. Bake for 30•40 minutes, until the apples are tender when pierced with a fork.

6. Remove from oven and drizzle the honey or maple syrup over the top of the apples, if using.

7. Serve the baked apples warm, spooning some of the cinnamon•flavored juices over the top.

These baked apples make a delicious and healthy 0 point dessert or snack. The cinnamon and nutmeg add wonderful flavor, and the honey or maple syrup is optional if you want a little extra sweetness. Enjoy!

34. Stir•fried bok choy with garlic

Ingredients:

• 1 lb bok choy, washed and chopped into 1•inch pieces
• 2 tbsp low•sodium soy sauce
• 1 tbsp rice vinegar
• 1 tsp sesame oil
• 2 cloves garlic, minced
• 1 tsp grated fresh ginger (optional)
• 1 tbsp water
• Salt and pepper to taste

Instructions:

1. In a small bowl, whisk together the soy sauce, rice vinegar, and sesame oil. Set aside.

2. Heat a large skillet or wok over medium•high heat. Add the minced garlic and grated ginger (if using) and cook for 30 seconds, stirring constantly, until fragrant.

3. Add the chopped bok choy and 1 tbsp of water to the pan. Stir•fry for 2•3 minutes, until the bok choy is tender•crisp.

4. Pour the soy sauce mixture over the bok choy and toss to coat evenly. Cook for 1 more minute.

5. Season with salt and pepper to taste.

6. Serve the stir•fried bok choy immediately, while hot.

This simple stir•fry is a great 0 point side dish or vegetarian main course. The bok choy cooks quickly and the garlic and soy sauce add tons of flavor. Enjoy!

35. Cauliflower crust pizza with vegetables

Ingredients:

Crust:
• 1 head of cauliflower, riced (about 3 cups riced)
• 1 egg, beaten
• 1/4 cup grated Parmesan cheese
• 1/2 tsp dried oregano
• 1/4 tsp garlic powder
• Salt and pepper to taste

Toppings:
• 1/2 cup marinara or pizza sauce
• 1 cup sliced mushrooms
• 1 cup chopped bell peppers
• 1/2 cup sliced onions
• 1 cup baby spinach leaves
• 1/2 cup shredded part•skim mozzarella cheese

Instructions:

1. Preheat oven to 400°F. Line a baking sheet with parchment paper.

2. Make the cauliflower crust: Pulse the cauliflower florets in a food processor until it resembles rice. Transfer to a microwave•safe bowl and microwave for 5 minutes. Allow to cool slightly.

3. In a bowl, mix the riced cauliflower, egg, Parmesan, oregano, garlic powder, salt and pepper until well combined.

4. Press the cauliflower mixture onto the prepared baking sheet, forming a thin round crust.

5. Bake the crust for 20•25 minutes until golden brown.

6. Top the baked crust with the marinara sauce, vegetables, and mozzarella cheese.

7. Bake for an additional 10•15 minutes until the cheese is melted and bubbly.

8. Slice and serve hot.

This cauliflower crust pizza is a delicious 0 point option for weight loss. The veggie•packed toppings make it a nutritious and satisfying meal.

36. Ratatouille

Ingredients:

- 1 medium eggplant, diced
- 1 medium zucchini, diced
- 1 medium yellow squash, diced
- 1 red bell pepper, diced
- 1 onion, diced
- 3 cloves garlic, minced
- 1 (14.5 oz) can diced tomatoes
- 2 tbsp olive oil
- 1 tsp dried thyme
- 1 tsp dried oregano
- Salt and pepper to taste
- Fresh basil leaves for garnish (optional)

Instructions:

1. In a large skillet or Dutch oven, heat the olive oil over medium heat. Add the diced eggplant, zucchini, squash, bell pepper, and onion. Sauté for 8·10 minutes, stirring occasionally, until the vegetables are tender.

2. Add the minced garlic and sauté for 1 minute more until fragrant.

3. Pour in the can of diced tomatoes along with the thyme, oregano, salt, and pepper. Stir to combine.

4. Reduce heat to low and let the ratatouille simmer for 15·20 minutes, stirring occasionally, until the flavors have melded and the vegetables are very tender.

5. Taste and adjust seasonings as needed.

6. Serve the ratatouille warm, garnished with fresh basil leaves if desired.

This classic French vegetable stew is a delicious 0 point dish for weight loss. It's packed with fiber, vitamins, and antioxidants from the variety of vegetables. Enjoy it as a main course or side dish.

37. Lemon garlic shrimp skewers

Ingredients:

- 1 lb large shrimp, peeled and deveined
- 2 tbsp olive oil
- 3 cloves garlic, minced
- 1 tbsp lemon juice
- 1 tsp lemon zest
- 1/4 tsp red pepper flakes (optional)
- Salt and pepper to taste
- Wooden or metal skewers

Instructions:

1. In a medium bowl, combine the shrimp, olive oil, minced garlic, lemon juice, lemon zest, and red pepper flakes (if using). Toss to coat the shrimp evenly. Season with salt and pepper.

2. Thread the shrimp onto skewers, leaving a little space between each one.

3. Preheat grill or grill pan to medium•high heat.

4. Grill the shrimp skewers for 2•3 minutes per side, until the shrimp are opaque and cooked through.

5. Serve the lemon garlic shrimp skewers immediately, garnished with extra lemon wedges if desired.

These shrimp skewers are a delicious 0 point option for weight loss. The lemon and garlic flavors pair perfectly with the juicy shrimp. You can serve them as an appetizer or main dish, alongside a fresh salad or roasted vegetables.

Enjoy this healthy and flavorful seafood dish!

38. Chickpea salad with cucumber and tomato

Ingredients:

• 1 (15 oz) can chickpeas, drained and rinsed
• 1 cup diced cucumber
• 1 cup diced tomatoes
• 1/4 cup diced red onion
• 2 tbsp chopped fresh parsley
• 2 tbsp lemon juice
• 1 tbsp olive oil
• 1 tsp Dijon mustard
• 1/4 tsp garlic powder
• Salt and pepper to taste

Instructions:

1. In a large bowl, combine the drained and rinsed chickpeas, diced cucumber, tomatoes, red onion, and chopped parsley.

2. In a small bowl, whisk together the lemon juice, olive oil, Dijon mustard, and garlic powder.

3. Pour the dressing over the chickpea salad and toss gently to coat.

4. Season with salt and pepper to taste.

5. Chill the salad in the refrigerator for at least 30 minutes to allow the flavors to blend.

6. Serve chilled or at room temperature.

This chickpea salad is a refreshing and nutritious 0 point dish. The combination of chickpeas, cucumber, tomato, and the tangy lemon•Dijon dressing makes it a delicious and filling option for weight loss. Enjoy it as a main dish or side salad.

39. Grilled eggplant with balsamic glaze

Ingredients:

- 1 medium eggplant, sliced into 1/2•inch thick rounds
- 2 tbsp olive oil
- 1/4 cup balsamic vinegar
- 2 tbsp honey
- 1 garlic clove, minced
- Salt and pepper to taste
- Fresh basil leaves for garnish (optional)

Instructions:

1. Preheat grill or grill pan to medium•high heat.

2. Brush the eggplant slices on both sides with the olive oil. Season with salt and pepper.

3. Grill the eggplant for 3•4 minutes per side, until tender and charred in spots.

4. In a small saucepan, combine the balsamic vinegar and honey. Bring to a simmer over medium heat and cook for 5•7 minutes, stirring occasionally, until thickened into a glaze.

5. Remove the saucepan from heat and stir in the minced garlic.

6. Arrange the grilled eggplant slices on a serving platter. Drizzle the balsamic glaze over the top.

7. Garnish with fresh basil leaves if desired.

8. Serve the grilled eggplant with balsamic glaze warm or at room temperature.

This simple grilled eggplant dish is a delicious 0 point option for weight loss. The balsamic glaze adds a sweet and tangy flavor that complements the smoky grilled eggplant perfectly. Enjoy as a side dish or light main course.

40. Spinach and feta stuffed mushrooms

Ingredients:

• 12 large mushrooms, stems removed and finely chopped
• 1 tbsp olive oil
• 1/4 cup finely chopped onion
• 2 cloves garlic, minced
• 1 cup fresh spinach, chopped
• 1/2 cup crumbled feta cheese
• 2 tbsp grated Parmesan cheese
• 1/4 tsp dried oregano
• Salt and pepper to taste

Instructions:

1. Preheat oven to 375°F. Clean the mushrooms and remove the stems, finely chopping the stems.

2. In a skillet, heat the olive oil over medium heat. Add the chopped mushroom stems, onion, and garlic. Sauté for 3•4 minutes until softened.

3. Add the chopped spinach and cook for 1•2 minutes until wilted. Remove from heat and let cool slightly.

4. In a bowl, mix the sautéed mushroom stem mixture with the feta cheese, Parmesan cheese, and oregano. Season with salt and pepper.

5. Stuff the mushroom caps evenly with the spinach and feta filling.

6. Arrange the stuffed mushrooms on a baking sheet.

7. Bake for 12•15 minutes, until the mushrooms are tender and the filling is hot.

8. Serve the spinach and feta stuffed mushrooms warm.

These stuffed mushrooms make a delicious appetizer or side dish. The combination of spinach, feta, and Parmesan creates a flavorful filling that complements the earthy mushrooms perfectly. Enjoy!

41. Jicama sticks with lime juice and chili powder

Ingredients:

- 1 medium jicama, peeled and cut into 1/4•inch thick sticks
- 2 tbsp fresh lime juice
- 1 tsp chili powder
- 1/4 tsp salt

Instructions:

1. Peel the jicama and cut it into 1/4•inch thick sticks or matchsticks.

2. In a large bowl, toss the jicama sticks with the lime juice, chili powder, and salt until evenly coated.

3. Serve the jicama sticks immediately, or refrigerate until ready to serve.

That's it! This simple snack or side dish is refreshing, crunchy, and full of flavor.

The jicama provides a nice crunch and mild, slightly sweet flavor that pairs perfectly with the tangy lime juice and spicy chili powder. The salt helps balance out the flavors.

Jicama is a great low•calorie, low•carb vegetable that's high in fiber and vitamin C. This recipe makes a healthy, 0 point snack or side dish that's perfect for weight loss.

Enjoy the jicama sticks on their own or alongside grilled meats, fish, or as part of a veggie platter. The bright, zesty flavors make them a refreshing and satisfying treat.

42. Asparagus with poached eggs

Ingredients:

• 1 lb asparagus, trimmed
• 4 large eggs
• 2 tbsp white vinegar
• Salt and pepper to taste

Instructions:

1. Bring a large pot of salted water to a boil. Add the asparagus and cook for 3•5 minutes, until tender•crisp. Drain and set aside.

2. Fill a shallow saucepan with 3•4 inches of water and bring to a gentle simmer. Add the white vinegar.

3. Crack each egg individually into a small ramekin or cup. Gently slide the eggs one at a time into the simmering water. Poach for 3•5 minutes, until the whites are set but the yolks are still runny.

4. Using a slotted spoon, carefully remove the poached eggs from the water and place them on top of the cooked asparagus.

5. Season the asparagus and eggs with salt and pepper to taste.

6. Serve the asparagus with poached eggs immediately, while the eggs are still warm.

This dish makes a delicious 0 point breakfast, brunch, or light meal. The tender asparagus pairs perfectly with the runny poached eggs. The vinegar helps the eggs hold their shape when poaching.

This is a simple, healthy, and satisfying option for weight loss. Enjoy!

43. Turkey meatballs in marinara sauce

Ingredients:

• 1 lb ground turkey
• 1/4 cup whole wheat breadcrumbs
• 2 tbsp grated Parmesan cheese
• 1 egg, lightly beaten
• 2 cloves garlic, minced
• 1 tsp dried oregano
• 1/2 tsp salt
• 1/4 tsp black pepper
• 1 (24 oz) jar marinara sauce

Instructions:

1. In a large bowl, combine the ground turkey, breadcrumbs, Parmesan, egg, garlic, oregano, salt, and pepper. Mix well until fully incorporated.

2. Roll the turkey mixture into 1•inch meatballs, making about 20•24 meatballs total.

3. In a large skillet or saucepan, bring the marinara sauce to a simmer over medium heat.

4. Carefully add the turkey meatballs to the simmering sauce. Cover and cook for 15•20 minutes, gently stirring occasionally, until the meatballs are cooked through.

5. Serve the turkey meatballs in marinara sauce over zucchini noodles, spaghetti squash, or whole wheat pasta.

6. Garnish with additional Parmesan cheese and fresh basil if desired.

These turkey meatballs are a delicious 0 point option for weight loss. The lean ground turkey keeps them low in calories, while the marinara sauce and Parmesan add tons of flavor. Enjoy this healthy and satisfying meal!

44. Green bean salad with vinaigrette

Ingredients:

• 1 lb fresh green beans, trimmed and cut into 1•inch pieces
• 2 tbsp olive oil
• 1 tbsp red wine vinegar
• 1 tsp Dijon mustard
• 1 tsp honey
• 1 clove garlic, minced
• Salt and pepper to taste
• 2 tbsp chopped fresh parsley

Instructions:

1. Bring a large pot of salted water to a boil. Add the cut green beans and cook for 3•5 minutes, until tender•crisp. Drain and rinse with cold water to stop the cooking.

2. In a small bowl, whisk together the olive oil, red wine vinegar, Dijon mustard, honey, and minced garlic. Season with salt and pepper.

3. In a large bowl, toss the cooked green beans with the vinaigrette until well coated.

4. Sprinkle the chopped fresh parsley over the top of the green bean salad.

5. Refrigerate for at least 30 minutes to allow the flavors to blend.

6. Serve the green bean salad chilled or at room temperature.

This fresh and flavorful green bean salad is a delicious 0 point side dish or light main course for weight loss. The tangy vinaigrette complements the crisp green beans perfectly. Feel free to add any other fresh veggies you have on hand.

Enjoy this healthy and satisfying green bean salad!

45. Baked pear with yogurt

Ingredients:

- 4 ripe but firm pears, halved and cored
- 1/4 cup water
- 1 tsp ground cinnamon
- 1/2 cup plain Greek yogurt
- 1 tbsp honey (optional)

Instructions:

1. Preheat oven to 375°F.

2. Place the pear halves cut·side up in a baking dish. Pour the water into the bottom of the dish.

3. Sprinkle the pears evenly with the ground cinnamon.

4. Bake for 20·25 minutes, until the pears are tender when pierced with a fork.

5. Remove the baked pears from the oven and let cool slightly.

6. Serve the warm pear halves with a dollop of plain Greek yogurt on top. Drizzle with a bit of honey if desired.

This simple baked pear dessert or snack is a delicious 0 point option for weight loss. The natural sweetness of the pears is enhanced by the cinnamon, and the creamy yogurt adds a nice contrast in texture and flavor.

The pears can be baked ahead of time and served warm or at room temperature. This makes a great healthy treat or light dessert. Enjoy!

46. Stuffed acorn squash with quinoa

Ingredients:

• 2 small acorn squash, halved and seeded
• 1 cup cooked quinoa
• 1 cup chopped kale or spinach
• 1/2 cup diced tomatoes
• 2 tbsp chopped fresh parsley
• 1 tbsp olive oil
• 1 clove garlic, minced
• Salt and pepper to taste

Instructions:

1. Preheat oven to 400°F. Place the acorn squash halves cut•side up on a baking sheet. Bake for 30•40 minutes, until tender when pierced with a fork.

2. In a medium bowl, combine the cooked quinoa, chopped kale/spinach, diced tomatoes, parsley, olive oil, and minced garlic. Season with salt and pepper.

3. Scoop the quinoa mixture evenly into the baked acorn squash halves.

4. Return the stuffed squash to the oven and bake for an additional 10•15 minutes, until the filling is hot.

5. Serve the stuffed acorn squash warm.

This stuffed acorn squash dish is a delicious and nutritious 0 point meal for weight loss. The quinoa, vegetables, and squash provide fiber, protein, and essential vitamins and minerals.

The natural sweetness of the roasted acorn squash pairs beautifully with the savory quinoa filling. This makes a satisfying vegetarian main course or side dish.

Enjoy this healthy and flavorful stuffed squash recipe!

47. Broccoli slaw with cranberries and almonds

Ingredients:

- 1 (12 oz) bag broccoli slaw mix
- 1/4 cup dried cranberries
- 2 tbsp sliced almonds
- 2 tbsp apple cider vinegar
- 1 tbsp olive oil
- 1 tsp Dijon mustard
- 1 tsp honey
- Salt and pepper to taste

Instructions:

1. In a large bowl, combine the broccoli slaw mix, dried cranberries, and sliced almonds.

2. In a small bowl, whisk together the apple cider vinegar, olive oil, Dijon mustard, and honey. Season with salt and pepper.

3. Pour the vinaigrette over the broccoli slaw mixture and toss to coat evenly.

4. Refrigerate the broccoli slaw for at least 30 minutes to allow the flavors to blend.

5. Serve the broccoli slaw chilled or at room temperature.

This broccoli slaw makes a delicious 0 point side dish or light main course for weight loss. The crunchy broccoli slaw, sweet cranberries, and toasted almonds create a wonderful texture and flavor combination.

The tangy vinaigrette ties all the ingredients together perfectly. This slaw is packed with fiber, vitamins, and antioxidants, making it a nutritious and satisfying option.

Enjoy this refreshing and flavorful broccoli slaw!

48. Cucumber cups with hummus

Ingredients:

• 1 large cucumber
• 1 cup prepared hummus
• 2 tbsp chopped fresh parsley or dill (optional)

Instructions:

1. Slice the cucumber into 1•inch thick rounds. Use a small spoon or melon baller to scoop out the center of each cucumber round, creating a small cup.

2. Fill each cucumber cup evenly with the prepared hummus.

3. Garnish the filled cucumber cups with the chopped fresh parsley or dill, if desired.

4. Arrange the cucumber cups on a serving platter and refrigerate until ready to serve.

That's it! This simple appetizer or snack is a delicious 0 point option for weight loss.

The cool, crunchy cucumber provides a nice contrast to the creamy, protein•packed hummus. The hummus adds flavor and nutrition without any extra points.

These cucumber cups are easy to make and perfect for entertaining or as a healthy on•the•go snack. You can use any variety of hummus • classic, roasted red pepper, garlic, etc.

Enjoy these refreshing and satisfying cucumber cups with hummus! They make a great low•calorie, low•carb option for weight loss.

49. Grilled pineapple skewers

Ingredients:

• 1 fresh pineapple, peeled, cored, and cut into 1•inch cubes
• 1 tbsp honey
• 1 tsp ground cinnamon
• Wooden or metal skewers

Instructions:

1. Preheat grill or grill pan to medium•high heat.

2. Thread the pineapple cubes onto the skewers, leaving a little space between each piece.

3. In a small bowl, mix together the honey and cinnamon.

4. Brush the pineapple skewers all over with the honey•cinnamon mixture.

5. Grill the pineapple skewers for 2•3 minutes per side, until lightly charred and caramelized.

6. Serve the grilled pineapple skewers warm.

These grilled pineapple skewers make a delicious 0 point dessert or snack for weight loss. The natural sweetness of the pineapple is enhanced by the honey and warm cinnamon flavors.

The grilling adds a nice caramelized, smoky flavor to the pineapple. These skewers are refreshing, juicy, and satisfying.

You can serve the grilled pineapple on its own or alongside grilled chicken or fish for a complete meal. Enjoy this healthy and flavorful summer treat!

50. Miso soup with tofu and seaweed

Ingredients:

• 4 cups low•sodium vegetable or chicken broth
• 2 tbsp white or yellow miso paste
• 1 block firm tofu, cut into 1•inch cubes
• 1 cup thinly sliced shiitake mushrooms
• 1/2 cup chopped wakame seaweed (or other dried seaweed)
• 2 green onions, thinly sliced
• 1 tsp sesame oil (optional)

Instructions:

1. In a medium saucepan, bring the broth to a gentle simmer over medium heat.

2. In a small bowl, whisk together the miso paste with a few tablespoons of the hot broth until smooth. Pour the miso mixture back into the saucepan, whisking to incorporate.

3. Add the cubed tofu, sliced shiitake mushrooms, and chopped wakame seaweed to the broth. Simmer for 2•3 minutes, until the seaweed has softened.

4. Remove the miso soup from heat and stir in the sliced green onions.

5. Ladle the miso soup into bowls and drizzle with sesame oil, if desired.

6. Serve the miso soup hot.

This miso soup is a delicious and nutritious 0 point option for weight loss. The miso paste provides umami flavor, while the tofu, mushrooms, and seaweed add protein, fiber, and essential vitamins and minerals.

Miso soup is a comforting and satisfying dish that can be enjoyed as a light meal or appetizer. Adjust the amount of miso paste to your desired saltiness and flavor.

Enjoy this healthy and flavorful miso soup!

51. Avocado salad with lime dressing

Ingredients:

- 2 ripe avocados, diced
- 1 cup cherry tomatoes, halved
- 1/2 red onion, thinly sliced
- 1/4 cup chopped fresh cilantro
- 2 tbsp lime juice
- 1 tbsp olive oil
- 1 tsp honey
- Salt and pepper to taste

Instructions:

1. In a large bowl, gently toss together the diced avocado, cherry tomatoes, red onion slices, and chopped cilantro.

2. In a small bowl, whisk together the lime juice, olive oil, and honey. Season with salt and pepper.

3. Pour the lime dressing over the avocado salad and toss gently to coat.

4. Serve the avocado salad immediately, or refrigerate for 30 minutes to allow the flavors to blend.

This avocado salad is a refreshing and nutritious 0 point dish for weight loss. The creamy avocado, juicy tomatoes, and tangy lime dressing create a delicious flavor combination.

The healthy fats from the avocado and the fiber from the vegetables make this salad very satisfying. It's perfect as a light main course or side dish.

Enjoy this simple yet flavorful avocado salad! It's a great way to incorporate more nutrient•dense ingredients into your diet.

52. Roasted beetroot with goat cheese

Ingredients:

- 3 medium beets, peeled and cut into 1•inch cubes
- 1 tbsp olive oil
- Salt and pepper to taste
- 2 oz crumbled goat cheese
- 2 tbsp chopped fresh parsley

Instructions:

1. Preheat oven to 400°F. Line a baking sheet with parchment paper.

2. In a bowl, toss the cubed beets with the olive oil. Season with salt and pepper.

3. Spread the beets in a single layer on the prepared baking sheet.

4. Roast the beets for 25•30 minutes, stirring halfway, until they are tender and lightly caramelized.

5. Remove the roasted beets from the oven and transfer to a serving bowl.

6. Sprinkle the crumbled goat cheese and chopped parsley over the top of the beets.

7. Serve the roasted beets with goat cheese warm or at room temperature.

This simple roasted beet dish is a delicious 0 point option for weight loss. The natural sweetness of the beets pairs beautifully with the tangy goat cheese.

The roasting brings out the beets' earthy, rich flavor. This makes a great side dish or light main course salad. You can also add other veggies like arugula or walnuts for extra nutrition.

Enjoy this flavorful and nutritious roasted beet recipe!

53. Baked sweet potato fries

Ingredients:

- 2 medium sweet potatoes, peeled and cut into 1/2•inch thick fry shapes
- 1 tbsp olive oil
- 1 tsp paprika
- 1/2 tsp garlic powder
- 1/4 tsp salt
- 1/4 tsp black pepper

Instructions:

1. Preheat oven to 400°F. Line a baking sheet with parchment paper.

2. In a large bowl, toss the sweet potato fry shapes with the olive oil, paprika, garlic powder, salt, and pepper until evenly coated.

3. Spread the seasoned sweet potato fries in a single layer on the prepared baking sheet.

4. Bake for 20•25 minutes, flipping the fries halfway through, until they are tender and lightly browned.

5. Remove the baked sweet potato fries from the oven and serve hot.

These baked sweet potato fries are a delicious 0 point side dish or snack for weight loss. The natural sweetness of the potatoes is enhanced by the spices, and baking them instead of frying keeps them low in calories.

Sweet potatoes are packed with fiber, vitamins, and antioxidants, making them a nutritious alternative to regular french fries. Enjoy these crispy, flavorful sweet potato fries as part of a healthy meal.

You can customize the seasonings to your taste • try adding cayenne, chili powder, or rosemary for different flavor variations.

54. Seared scallops with mango salsa

Ingredients:

Mango Salsa:
- 1 ripe mango, diced
- 1/2 red onion, finely chopped
- 1 jalapeño, seeded and minced
- 2 tbsp chopped fresh cilantro
- 1 tbsp lime juice
- Salt and pepper to taste

Scallops:
- 1 lb sea scallops, patted dry
- 1 tbsp olive oil
- Salt and pepper to taste

Instructions:

1. Make the mango salsa: In a medium bowl, combine the diced mango, red onion, jalapeño, cilantro, and lime juice. Season with salt and pepper to taste. Set aside.

2. Pat the scallops very dry with paper towels and season with salt and pepper.

3. Heat the olive oil in a large skillet over high heat. When the oil is shimmering, add the scallops in a single layer, making sure not to overcrowd the pan.

4. Sear the scallops for 2•3 minutes per side, until a nice golden•brown crust forms and the centers are opaque.

5. Transfer the seared scallops to a plate.

6. Serve the hot scallops immediately, topped with the fresh mango salsa.

The sweet and tangy mango salsa provides a delicious contrast to the caramelized, savory scallops. This dish makes a beautiful and flavorful appetizer or light main course.

Enjoy the bright, tropical flavors of this seared scallops with mango salsa recipe!

55. Quinoa stuffed bell peppers

Ingredients:

• 4 bell peppers, halved lengthwise and seeded
• 1 cup cooked quinoa
• 1 cup diced tomatoes
• 1/2 cup canned black beans, rinsed and drained
• 1/4 cup diced onion
• 2 cloves garlic, minced
• 1 tsp chili powder
• 1/2 tsp cumin
• Salt and pepper to taste
• 2 tbsp crumbled feta cheese (optional)

Instructions:

1. Preheat oven to 375°F. Place the bell pepper halves cut•side up in a baking dish.

2. In a medium bowl, mix together the cooked quinoa, diced tomatoes, black beans, onion, garlic, chili powder, cumin, salt, and pepper.

3. Spoon the quinoa mixture evenly into the bell pepper halves.

4. Cover the baking dish with foil and bake for 25•30 minutes, until the peppers are tender.

5. Remove the foil and sprinkle the stuffed peppers with the crumbled feta cheese, if using.

6. Return the dish to the oven and bake for an additional 5 minutes.

7. Serve the quinoa stuffed bell peppers warm.

These quinoa stuffed bell peppers are a delicious and nutritious 0 point meal for weight loss. The quinoa provides fiber and protein, while the bell peppers and other veggies add vitamins, minerals, and antioxidants.

The feta cheese is optional, but it adds a nice tangy flavor. You can also customize the filling with other vegetables, herbs, or spices to your taste.

Enjoy this healthy and satisfying stuffed pepper dish!

56. Carrot and ginger soup

Ingredients:

- 1 lb carrots, peeled and chopped
- 1 onion, diced
- 2 cloves garlic, minced
- 1 tbsp grated fresh ginger
- 4 cups low•sodium vegetable or chicken broth
- 1 tsp ground cumin
- 1/4 tsp cayenne pepper (optional)
- Salt and pepper to taste
- Chopped fresh parsley for garnish (optional)

Instructions:

1. In a large pot or Dutch oven, sauté the chopped onion in a small amount of broth or water over medium heat for 3•4 minutes until translucent.

2. Add the minced garlic and grated ginger. Cook for 1 minute, stirring constantly, until fragrant.

3. Add the chopped carrots and vegetable/chicken broth. Bring the soup to a boil.

4. Reduce heat to low, cover, and simmer for 20•25 minutes, until the carrots are very tender.

5. Using an immersion blender, carefully blend the soup until smooth and creamy.

6. Stir in the ground cumin and cayenne pepper (if using). Season with salt and pepper to taste.

7. Ladle the carrot ginger soup into bowls and garnish with chopped fresh parsley, if desired.

This carrot and ginger soup is a delicious 0 point option for weight loss. The carrots provide fiber, vitamins, and natural sweetness, while the ginger adds a nice warmth and zing.

The soup is creamy and comforting, yet low in calories. Serve it as a starter or light main course. Enjoy!

57. Turkey lettuce cups with hoisin sauce

Ingredients:

• 1 lb ground turkey
• 2 cloves garlic, minced
• 1 tbsp grated fresh ginger
• 2 tbsp low•sodium soy sauce
• 1 tbsp rice vinegar
• 1 tbsp hoisin sauce
• 1 tsp sesame oil
• 1/4 tsp red pepper flakes (optional)
• 8•10 large lettuce leaves (such as bibb or romaine)
• Chopped green onions, for garnish

Instructions:

1. In a large skillet or wok, cook the ground turkey over medium•high heat, breaking it up with a wooden spoon, until browned and cooked through, about 5•7 minutes.

2. Add the minced garlic and grated ginger to the skillet. Cook for 1 minute, until fragrant.

3. Stir in the soy sauce, rice vinegar, hoisin sauce, sesame oil, and red pepper flakes (if using). Toss to coat the turkey mixture.

4. Spoon the turkey mixture into the lettuce leaves.

5. Top the turkey lettuce cups with chopped green onions.

6. Serve immediately.

These turkey lettuce cups are a delicious 0 point meal or appetizer for weight loss. The lean ground turkey is flavored with savory hoisin sauce, garlic, and ginger. The cool, crisp lettuce leaves provide a nice contrast.

This recipe is easy to make and perfect for a healthy, low•carb meal. You can customize the filling with other veggies or herbs as well. Enjoy these flavorful turkey lettuce cups!

58. Kale salad with lemon tahini dressing

Ingredients:

Salad:
• 1 bunch kale, stems removed and leaves chopped
• 1 cup shredded carrots
• 1/2 cup diced cucumber
• 1/4 cup toasted sliced almonds

Lemon Tahini Dressing:
• 2 tbsp tahini
• 2 tbsp lemon juice
• 1 tbsp water
• 1 tsp honey
• 1 clove garlic, minced
• Salt and pepper to taste

Instructions:

1. In a large bowl, combine the chopped kale, shredded carrots, diced cucumber, and toasted almonds.

2. In a small bowl, whisk together the tahini, lemon juice, water, honey, and minced garlic. Season with salt and pepper.

3. Pour the lemon tahini dressing over the kale salad and toss to coat evenly.

4. Let the salad sit for 5•10 minutes to allow the kale to soften slightly.

5. Serve the kale salad chilled or at room temperature.

This kale salad with lemon tahini dressing is a delicious and nutritious 0 point option for weight loss. The massaged kale provides fiber and vitamins, while the tahini dressing adds healthy fats and creaminess.

The bright lemon flavor and crunch of the almonds make this salad incredibly satisfying. It's a great side dish or light main course.

Feel free to add other veggies, fruits, or proteins to customize this kale salad to your liking. Enjoy this healthy and flavorful dish!

59. Cauliflower steaks with chimichurri sauce

Ingredients:

Cauliflower Steaks:
• 1 large head of cauliflower, cut into 1•inch thick slices
• 2 tbsp olive oil
• Salt and pepper to taste

Chimichurri Sauce:
• 1 cup packed fresh parsley leaves
• 3 cloves garlic
• 2 tbsp red wine vinegar
• 1 tbsp olive oil
• 1 tsp dried oregano
• 1/4 tsp red pepper flakes
• Salt and pepper to taste

Instructions:

1. Make the chimichurri sauce: In a food processor, combine the parsley, garlic, red wine vinegar, olive oil, oregano, and red pepper flakes. Pulse until a coarse sauce forms. Season with salt and pepper to taste. Set aside.

2. Preheat oven to 400°F. Line a baking sheet with parchment paper.

3. Brush the cauliflower slices on both sides with the 2 tbsp of olive oil. Season generously with salt and pepper.

4. Arrange the cauliflower steaks in a single layer on the prepared baking sheet.

5. Roast the cauliflower for 20•25 minutes, flipping halfway, until tender and lightly browned.

6. Transfer the roasted cauliflower steaks to a serving plate. Drizzle the chimichurri sauce generously over the top.

7. Serve the cauliflower steaks with chimichurri immediately, while hot.

The bold, herby chimichurri sauce complements the tender, caramelized cauliflower steaks perfectly in this dish. It makes a delicious vegetarian main course or side.

The cauliflower provides fiber, vitamins, and minerals, while the chimichurri adds healthy fats and tons of flavor. Enjoy this simple yet impressive recipe!

60. Baked cod with tomatoes and olives

Ingredients:

• 1 lb cod fillets
• 1 (14.5 oz) can diced tomatoes
• 1/2 cup pitted kalamata olives, halved
• 2 cloves garlic, minced
• 1 tbsp olive oil
• 1 tsp dried oregano
• Salt and pepper to taste
• Chopped fresh parsley for garnish (optional)

Instructions:

1. Preheat oven to 400°F. Lightly grease a baking dish.

2. Place the cod fillets In the prepared baking dish.

3. In a bowl, mix together the diced tomatoes, olives, minced garlic, olive oil, and dried oregano. Season with salt and pepper.

4. Spoon the tomato•olive mixture over and around the cod fillets.

5. Bake for 15•20 minutes, until the cod is opaque and flakes easily with a fork.

6. Garnish the baked cod with chopped fresh parsley, if desired.

7. Serve the cod immediately, with the tomato•olive sauce spooned over the top.

This baked cod dish is a delicious and healthy 0 point option for weight loss. The tomatoes and olives provide a flavorful Mediterranean•inspired topping for the tender, flaky cod.

The simple preparation allows the natural flavors of the fish and vegetables to shine. Serve this baked cod with a side of roasted vegetables or a fresh salad for a complete and satisfying meal.

Enjoy this easy and nutritious seafood recipe!

61. Radish and cucumber salad

Ingredients:

- 1 bunch radishes, thinly sliced
- 1 English cucumber, thinly sliced
- 1/4 red onion, thinly sliced
- 2 tbsp rice vinegar
- 1 tbsp olive oil
- 1 tsp Dijon mustard
- 1 tsp honey
- 2 tbsp chopped fresh dill
- Salt and pepper to taste

Instructions:

1. In a large bowl, combine the thinly sliced radishes, cucumber, and red onion.

2. In a small bowl, whisk together the rice vinegar, olive oil, Dijon mustard, and honey. Season with salt and pepper.

3. Pour the vinaigrette over the radish and cucumber salad and toss gently to coat.

4. Sprinkle the chopped fresh dill over the top of the salad.

5. Refrigerate the salad for at least 30 minutes to allow the flavors to blend.

6. Serve the radish and cucumber salad chilled or at room temperature.

This refreshing salad is a delicious 0 point option for weight loss. The crunchy radishes and cucumbers provide a satisfying texture, while the tangy vinaigrette and fresh dill add tons of flavor.

The salad is hydrating, low in calories, and packed with vitamins and minerals. It makes a great side dish or light main course.

Feel free to add other veggies like bell peppers or cherry tomatoes to customize the salad. Enjoy this simple yet flavorful radish and cucumber salad!

62. Grilled vegetable kebabs

Ingredients:

• 1 zucchini, cut into 1•inch chunks
• 1 yellow squash, cut into 1•inch chunks
• 1 red bell pepper, cut into 1•inch pieces
• 1 red onion, cut into 1•inch pieces
• 8 oz mushrooms, halved
• 2 tbsp olive oil
• 1 tsp dried oregano
• 1/2 tsp garlic powder
• Salt and pepper to taste

Instructions:

1. Preheat grill or grill pan to medium•high heat.

2. In a large bowl, toss the chopped vegetables with the olive oil, oregano, garlic powder, salt, and pepper until evenly coated.

3. Thread the seasoned vegetables onto skewers, alternating the different veggies.

4. Grill the vegetable kebabs for 12•15 minutes, turning occasionally, until the vegetables are tender and lightly charred.

5. Serve the grilled vegetable kebabs immediately, while hot.

These grilled vegetable kebabs are a delicious 0 point option for weight loss. The combination of zucchini, squash, bell pepper, onion, and mushrooms provides a variety of nutrients and flavors.

The high•heat grilling caramelizes the natural sugars in the veggies, adding a wonderful smoky, roasted taste. You can use any combination of your favorite grillable vegetables.

Serve the kebabs as a main dish or side. They pair well with grilled chicken, fish, or tofu for a complete meal. Enjoy this healthy and flavorful summer recipe!

63. Tofu stir•fry with broccoli

Ingredients:

• 1 block extra•firm tofu, pressed and cubed
• 2 cups broccoli florets
• 1 tbsp low•sodium soy sauce
• 1 tbsp rice vinegar
• 1 tsp sesame oil
• 1 tsp honey
• 2 cloves garlic, minced
• 1 tsp grated fresh ginger
• 1 tbsp water
• Salt and pepper to taste
• Chopped green onions for garnish (optional)

Instructions:

1. In a small bowl, whisk together the soy sauce, rice vinegar, sesame oil, and honey. Set aside.

2. Heat a large non•stick skillet or wok over medium•high heat. Add the cubed tofu and cook for 3•4 minutes per side, until lightly browned. Transfer the tofu to a plate.

3. Add the broccoli florets and 1 tbsp of water to the skillet. Cover and steam for 2•3 minutes, until the broccoli is tender•crisp.

4. Push the broccoli to the side of the skillet. Add the minced garlic and grated ginger to the center of the pan. Cook for 1 minute, until fragrant.

5. Add the cooked tofu back to the skillet. Pour in the soy sauce mixture and toss everything together until well coated.

6. Cook for 2•3 minutes more, until the sauce has thickened slightly.

7. Serve the tofu stir•fry with broccoli immediately, garnished with chopped green onions if desired.

This tofu and broccoli stir•fry is a delicious and nutritious 0 point meal for weight loss. The high•protein tofu and fiber•rich broccoli make it a satisfying vegetarian dish.

The simple sauce adds tons of flavor without any extra points. Serve it over steamed rice or cauliflower rice for a complete meal.

64. Melon gazpacho

Ingredients:

• 4 cups diced ripe cantaloupe or honeydew melon
• 1 cup diced cucumber
• 1/2 cup diced red onion
• 2 tablespoons chopped fresh mint
• 2 tablespoons chopped fresh cilantro
• 2 tablespoons lime juice
• 1 tablespoon sherry vinegar or white wine vinegar
• 1/4 teaspoon salt
• Freshly ground black pepper to taste

Instructions:

1. In a large bowl, combine the diced melon, cucumber, red onion, mint, cilantro, lime juice, vinegar, salt and pepper. Stir gently to combine.

2. Cover and refrigerate for at least 30 minutes to allow the flavors to meld.

3. Serve chilled, in bowls or glasses. Top with additional mint or cilantro if desired.

This refreshing cold soup makes a great starter or light main course on a hot summer day. The sweet melon pairs nicely with the tangy vinegar and fresh herbs. Adjust the seasoning to your taste. Enjoy!

65. Eggplant rollatini

Ingredients:

• 2 medium eggplants, sliced lengthwise into 1/4•inch thick slices
• 1 cup part•skim ricotta cheese
• 1 cup shredded part•skim mozzarella cheese
• 1/4 cup grated Parmesan cheese
• 1 egg, lightly beaten
• 2 tablespoons chopped fresh parsley
• 1 teaspoon dried oregano
• 1/4 teaspoon salt
• 1/4 teaspoon black pepper
• 1 cup marinara sauce

Instructions:

1. Preheat oven to 375°F. Lightly grease a baking sheet.

2. Arrange the eggplant slices in a single layer on the prepared baking sheet. Bake for 10•12 minutes, flipping halfway, until softened and pliable.

3. In a medium bowl, mix together the ricotta, 1/2 cup of the mozzarella, Parmesan, egg, parsley, oregano, salt and pepper.

4. Spread 2•3 tablespoons of the ricotta mixture onto each eggplant slice. Carefully roll up the slices and place seam•side down in a baking dish.

5. Top the rolled eggplant with the marinara sauce and remaining 1/2 cup mozzarella cheese.

6. Bake for 20•25 minutes, until heated through and cheese is melted.

7. Let stand 5 minutes before serving.

This eggplant rollatini dish is delicious but higher in calories and fat, so it would not be considered a weight loss•friendly recipe. The combination of the breaded and fried eggplant, cheese, and sauce makes it a richer, more indulgent dish.

66. Greek yogurt with honey and walnuts

Ingredients:

• 1 cup plain Greek yogurt
• 1•2 tablespoons honey
• 2 tablespoons chopped walnuts

Instructions:

1. Spoon the Greek yogurt into a bowl.

2. Drizzle the honey over the top.

3. Sprinkle the chopped walnuts over the honey.

Nutritional Information:

• Calories: Approximately 200•250 calories

• This dish would not be considered 0 points for weight loss, as the combination of the Greek yogurt, honey, and walnuts provides a significant amount of calories and fat.

While Greek yogurt, honey, and walnuts are all nutritious ingredients, this particular dish is higher in calories and fat compared to other snack or breakfast options that may be more weight loss•friendly. The honey and walnuts add a significant amount of calories and fat that should be accounted for in a weight loss plan.

67. Stuffed cabbage rolls with lean ground beef

Ingredients:

- 1 lb lean ground beef
- 1 cup cooked brown rice
- 1 onion, finely chopped
- 2 cloves garlic, minced
- 1 tsp dried oregano
- Salt and pepper to taste
- 1 large head of green cabbage
- 1 (15 oz) can tomato sauce
- 1 (15 oz) can diced tomatoes

Instructions:

1. In a bowl, mix together the ground beef, cooked rice, onion, garlic, oregano, salt, and pepper.

2. Core the cabbage and carefully remove the leaves, keeping them intact.

3. Place a spoonful of the beef mixture onto each cabbage leaf and roll up, tucking in the sides.

4. Arrange the stuffed cabbage rolls in a baking dish. Pour the tomato sauce and diced tomatoes over the top.

5. Bake at 375°F for 45•60 minutes, until the cabbage is tender and the filling is cooked through.

Nutritional Information:
- Calories: Approximately 300•400 calories per serving
- This dish would not be considered 0 points for weight loss, as the combination of the ground beef, rice, and tomato sauce provides a significant amount of calories and carbohydrates.

While the use of lean ground beef and the inclusion of vegetables like cabbage make this a relatively healthy dish, the overall calorie and carbohydrate content would not make it an ideal choice for a weight loss plan. The portion size and frequency of consumption would need to be carefully monitored.

68. Roasted kabocha squash

Ingredients:

• 1 medium kabocha squash, peeled, seeded, and cut into 1•inch cubes
• 1 tbsp olive oil
• Salt and pepper to taste

Instructions:
1. Preheat the oven to 400°F.

2. Toss the cubed kabocha squash with the olive oil, salt, and pepper in a large bowl.

3. Spread the squash cubes in a single layer on a baking sheet.

4. Roast for 25•30 minutes, flipping halfway, until the squash is tender and lightly browned.

Nutritional Information:

• Calories: Approximately 100•150 calories per 1 cup serving

• This dish would not be considered 0 points for weight loss, as the natural sugars and carbohydrates in the kabocha squash contribute to the overall calorie content.

While kabocha squash is a nutrient•dense, low•calorie vegetable, it is still a source of carbohydrates and calories. The roasting process can also concentrate the natural sugars, making it a bit higher in calories compared to some other non•starchy vegetables.

For a weight loss plan, roasted kabocha squash can be a healthy and satisfying side dish, but the portion size should be monitored to fit within your daily calorie and carbohydrate goals.

69. Tomato basil bruschetta

Ingredients:

• 1 baguette, sliced into 1/2•inch thick rounds
• 3 tomatoes, diced
• 1/4 cup fresh basil leaves, chopped
• 2 cloves garlic, minced
• 2 tbsp olive oil
• 1 tbsp balsamic vinegar
• Salt and pepper to taste

Instructions:

1. Preheat the oven to 400°F.

2. Arrange the baguette slices on a baking sheet and toast in the oven for 5•7 minutes, until lightly golden.

3. In a bowl, combine the diced tomatoes, chopped basil, garlic, olive oil, and balsamic vinegar. Season with salt and pepper.

4. Top the toasted baguette slices with the tomato basil mixture.

Nutritional Information:
• Calories: Approximately 100•150 calories per serving (2•3 bruschetta)

• This dish would not be considered 0 points for weight loss, as the combination of the bread, olive oil, and balsamic vinegar contributes a significant amount of calories and carbohydrates.

While the tomatoes and basil provide nutritional benefits, the overall calorie and carbohydrate content of the bruschetta makes it a less ideal choice for a weight loss plan. The portion size and frequency of consumption would need to be carefully monitored to fit within your daily calorie and macronutrient goals.

70. Cucumber avocado gazpacho

Ingredients:

- 2 cups diced cucumber
- 1 ripe avocado, pitted and diced
- 1/2 cup plain Greek yogurt
- 1/4 cup fresh cilantro, chopped
- 2 tbsp lime juice
- 1 clove garlic, minced
- 1/4 tsp salt
- 1/4 tsp black pepper

Instructions:

1. In a blender or food processor, combine the diced cucumber, avocado, Greek yogurt, cilantro, lime juice, garlic, salt, and pepper.

2. Blend until smooth and creamy.

3. Chill the gazpacho in the refrigerator for at least 30 minutes before serving.

Nutritional Information:
- Calories: Approximately 150•200 calories per serving

- This dish would not be considered 0 points for weight loss, as the combination of the avocado and Greek yogurt contributes a significant amount of calories and fat.

While the cucumber, avocado, and other ingredients provide nutritional benefits, the overall calorie and fat content of the gazpacho would need to be considered in a weight loss plan. The portion size and frequency of consumption would need to be carefully monitored to fit within your daily calorie and macronutrient goals.

71. Broccoli and quinoa casserole

Ingredients:

• 1 cup uncooked quinoa, rinsed
• 2 cups low•sodium vegetable or chicken broth
• 2 cups chopped broccoli florets
• 1/2 cup shredded cheddar cheese
• 2 eggs, lightly beaten
• 1/4 cup plain Greek yogurt
• 1 clove garlic, minced
• 1/4 tsp salt
• 1/4 tsp black pepper

Instructions:

1. Preheat the oven to 375°F. Grease a 9x9•inch baking dish.

2. In a saucepan, combine the quinoa and broth. Bring to a boil, then reduce heat and simmer for 15•20 minutes, until quinoa is cooked.

3. In a large bowl, mix the cooked quinoa, broccoli, cheddar cheese, eggs, Greek yogurt, garlic, salt, and pepper.

4. Transfer the mixture to the prepared baking dish and spread evenly.

5. Bake for 25•30 minutes, until the casserole is set and the top is lightly browned.

Nutritional Information:
• Calories: Approximately 250•300 calories per serving

• This dish would not be considered 0 points for weight loss, as the combination of the quinoa, cheese, and eggs contributes a moderate amount of calories and macronutrients.

While the broccoli and quinoa provide nutritional benefits, the overall calorie and macronutrient content of the casserole would need to be considered in a weight loss plan. The portion size and frequency of consumption would need to be carefully monitored to fit within your daily calorie and macronutrient goals.

72. Turkey and vegetable skewers

Ingredients:

• 1 lb boneless, skinless turkey breast, cut into 1•inch cubes
• 1 red bell pepper, cut into 1•inch pieces
• 1 zucchini, cut into 1•inch pieces
• 1 red onion, cut into 1•inch pieces
• 2 tbsp olive oil
• 1 tsp dried oregano
• Salt and pepper to taste

Instructions:

1. Preheat grill or grill pan to medium•high heat.

2. Thread the turkey cubes, bell pepper, zucchini, and onion pieces onto skewers.

3. Brush the skewers with the olive oil and sprinkle with the dried oregano, salt, and pepper.

4. Grill the skewers for 12•15 minutes, turning occasionally, until the turkey is cooked through and the vegetables are tender.

Nutritional Information:

• Calories: Approximately 150•200 calories per serving (2•3 skewers)

• This dish would not be considered 0 points for weight loss, as the combination of the turkey, vegetables, and olive oil contributes a moderate amount of calories and fat.

While the turkey and vegetables are generally healthy, low•calorie ingredients, the use of olive oil and the overall portion size of the skewers would need to be considered in a weight loss plan. The calorie and macronutrient content is still relatively moderate, making this a reasonably healthy option, but not necessarily a 0 point dish for weight loss.

73. Mango cucumber salad

Ingredients:

- 1 ripe mango, peeled and diced
- 1 cucumber, peeled, seeded, and diced
- 1/4 cup diced red onion
- 2 tbsp chopped fresh cilantro
- 1 tbsp lime juice
- 1 tsp honey
- 1/4 tsp salt
- 1/4 tsp black pepper

Instructions:

1. In a bowl, combine the diced mango, cucumber, red onion, and cilantro.

2. In a small bowl, whisk together the lime juice, honey, salt, and pepper.

3. Pour the dressing over the salad and toss gently to coat.

4. Chill the salad in the refrigerator for at least 30 minutes before serving.

Nutritional Information:

- Calories: Approximately 100•150 calories per serving

- This dish would not be considered 0 points for weight loss, as the combination of the mango and the dressing contributes a moderate amount of calories and natural sugars.

While the mango, cucumber, and other ingredients provide nutritional benefits, the overall calorie and carbohydrate content of the salad would need to be considered in a weight loss plan. The portion size and frequency of consumption would need to be carefully monitored to fit within your daily calorie and macronutrient goals.

74. Spaghetti squash with marinara

Ingredients:

• 1 medium spaghetti squash, halved lengthwise and seeded
• 1 cup marinara sauce
• 2 tbsp grated Parmesan cheese (optional)
• Fresh basil, chopped (optional)

Instructions:
1. Preheat the oven to 400°F.

2. Place the spaghetti squash halves cut•side down on a baking sheet. Bake for 40•50 minutes, until the squash is tender and easily shreds with a fork.

3. Remove the squash from the oven and let cool slightly. Use a fork to shred the flesh into spaghetti•like strands.

4. In a bowl, combine the shredded spaghetti squash with the marinara sauce. Toss to coat.

5. Serve the spaghetti squash with marinara, topped with Parmesan cheese and fresh basil, if desired.

Nutritional Information:
• Calories: Approximately 150•200 calories per serving

• This dish would not be considered 0 points for weight loss, as the combination of the spaghetti squash and marinara sauce contributes a moderate amount of calories and carbohydrates.

While spaghetti squash is a low•calorie, nutrient•dense vegetable, the addition of the marinara sauce adds some calories and carbohydrates. For a weight loss plan, the portion size and frequency of consumption would need to be carefully monitored to fit within your daily calorie and macronutrient goals.

75. Artichoke and spinach dip (lightened version)

Ingredients:

- 1 (14 oz) can artichoke hearts, drained and chopped
- 1 (10 oz) package frozen chopped spinach, thawed and squeezed dry
- 1/2 cup plain Greek yogurt
- 1/2 cup low•fat mayonnaise
- 1/2 cup shredded part•skim mozzarella cheese
- 1/4 cup grated Parmesan cheese
- 2 cloves garlic, minced
- 1/4 tsp red pepper flakes (optional)
- Salt and pepper to taste

Instructions:

1. Preheat the oven to 375°F.

2. In a bowl, mix together the chopped artichoke hearts, spinach, Greek yogurt, low•fat mayonnaise, mozzarella cheese, Parmesan cheese, garlic, and red pepper flakes (if using). Season with salt and pepper.

3. Transfer the dip mixture to a baking dish and smooth the top.

4. Bake for 20•25 minutes, until heated through and the top is lightly browned.

5. Serve warm with whole grain crackers, pita chips, or vegetable sticks.

Nutritional Information:

- Calories: Approximately 150•200 calories per serving

- This lightened version of the artichoke and spinach dip would not be considered 0 points for weight loss, as the combination of the dairy products and cheese still contributes a significant amount of calories and fat.

While this recipe uses lower•fat and healthier ingredients compared to a traditional artichoke and spinach dip, it is still a relatively high•calorie dish due to the cheese and dairy components. For a weight loss plan, the portion size and frequency of consumption would need to be carefully monitored to fit within your daily calorie and macronutrient goals.

76. Greek chicken skewers with tzatziki

Ingredients:

Chicken Skewers:
• 1 lb boneless, skinless chicken breasts, cut into 1•inch cubes
• 2 tbsp olive oil
• 2 tbsp lemon juice
• 1 tsp dried oregano
• 1 tsp garlic powder
• Salt and pepper to taste

Tzatziki Sauce:
• 1 cup plain Greek yogurt
• 1/2 cucumber, grated and squeezed dry
• 1 clove garlic, minced
• 1 tbsp lemon juice
• 1 tbsp chopped fresh dill
• 1/4 tsp salt

Instructions:

1. In a bowl, combine the chicken cubes, olive oil, lemon juice, oregano, garlic powder, salt, and pepper. Toss to coat.

2. Thread the chicken onto skewers.

3. In a separate bowl, mix together all the tzatziki sauce ingredients.

4. Grill the chicken skewers for 12•15 minutes, turning occasionally, until cooked through.

5. Serve the grilled chicken skewers with the tzatziki sauce.

Nutritional Information:
• Calories: Approximately 250•300 calories per serving (2•3 skewers with tzatziki)
• This dish would not be considered 0 points for weight loss, as the combination of the chicken, olive oil, and tzatziki sauce contributes a moderate amount of calories and fat.

While the chicken and vegetables provide nutritional benefits, the overall calorie and macronutrient content of the dish would need to be considered in a weight loss plan. The portion size and frequency of consumption would need to be carefully monitored to fit within your daily calorie and macronutrient goals.

77. Apple walnut salad with vinaigrette

Ingredients:

- 5 cups mixed greens (e.g., spinach, arugula, kale)
- 1 apple, diced
- 1/4 cup chopped walnuts
- 2 tbsp crumbled feta cheese
- 2 tbsp olive oil
- 1 tbsp apple cider vinegar
- 1 tsp Dijon mustard
- 1 tsp honey
- Salt and pepper to taste

Instructions:

1. In a large bowl, combine the mixed greens, diced apple, chopped walnuts, and crumbled feta cheese.

2. In a small bowl, whisk together the olive oil, apple cider vinegar, Dijon mustard, and honey. Season with salt and pepper.

3. Drizzle the vinaigrette over the salad and toss gently to coat.

Nutritional Information:

- Calories: Approximately 200•250 calories per serving

- This dish would not be considered 0 points for weight loss, as the combination of the olive oil, walnuts, and feta cheese contributes a significant amount of calories and fat.

While the salad itself is made up of nutrient•dense ingredients like greens, apples, and walnuts, the addition of the vinaigrette and cheese increases the overall calorie and fat content. For a weight loss plan, the portion size and frequency of consumption would need to be carefully monitored to fit within your daily calorie and macronutrient goals.

78. Roasted cauliflower with tahini sauce

Ingredients:

Roasted Cauliflower:
• 1 head of cauliflower, cut into florets
• 2 tbsp olive oil
• Salt and pepper to taste

Tahini Sauce:
• 1/4 cup tahini
• 2 tbsp lemon juice
• 1 clove garlic, minced
• 2•3 tbsp water
• Salt and pepper to taste

Instructions:
1. Preheat the oven to 400°F. Toss the cauliflower florets with the olive oil, salt, and pepper.

2. Spread the cauliflower on a baking sheet and roast for 20•25 minutes, until tender and lightly browned.

3. In a small bowl, whisk together the tahini, lemon juice, garlic, and 2•3 tbsp of water to create a smooth sauce. Season with salt and pepper.

4. Drizzle the tahini sauce over the roasted cauliflower and serve.

Nutritional Information:

• Calories: Approximately 200•250 calories per serving

• This dish would not be considered 0 points for weight loss, as the combination of the roasted cauliflower and the tahini sauce contributes a moderate amount of calories and fat.

While the cauliflower is a low•calorie, nutrient•dense vegetable, the tahini sauce adds a significant amount of calories and fat from the tahini. For a weight loss plan, the portion size and frequency of consumption would need to be carefully monitored to fit within your daily calorie and macronutrient goals.

79. Shrimp and avocado salad

Ingredients:

- 1 lb cooked shrimp, peeled and deveined
- 1 avocado, diced
- 1/2 cup diced cucumber
- 1/4 cup diced red onion
- 2 tbsp chopped fresh cilantro
- 2 tbsp lime juice
- 1 tbsp olive oil
- 1/4 tsp salt
- 1/4 tsp black pepper

Instructions:

1. In a large bowl, combine the cooked shrimp, diced avocado, cucumber, red onion, and chopped cilantro.

2. In a small bowl, whisk together the lime juice, olive oil, salt, and pepper.

3. Drizzle the dressing over the shrimp and avocado salad and toss gently to coat.

4. Serve chilled or at room temperature.

Nutritional Information:
• Calories: Approximately 250•300 calories per serving

• This dish would not be considered 0 points for weight loss, as the combination of the shrimp, avocado, and olive oil contributes a significant amount of calories and fat.

While the shrimp and avocado provide nutritional benefits, the overall calorie and fat content of the salad would need to be considered in a weight loss plan. The portion size and frequency of consumption would need to be carefully monitored to fit within your daily calorie and macronutrient goals.

80. Quinoa•stuffed mushrooms

Ingredients:

• 12 large mushrooms, stems removed and finely chopped
• 1/2 cup cooked quinoa
• 2 tbsp grated Parmesan cheese
• 2 tbsp panko breadcrumbs
• 1 tbsp olive oil
• 1 clove garlic, minced
• 1 tbsp chopped fresh parsley
• Salt and pepper to taste

Instructions:

1. Preheat the oven to 375°F. Lightly grease a baking sheet.

2. In a bowl, mix together the chopped mushroom stems, cooked quinoa, Parmesan cheese, panko breadcrumbs, olive oil, garlic, and parsley. Season with salt and pepper.

3. Stuff the mushroom caps with the quinoa mixture, packing it in gently.

4. Arrange the stuffed mushrooms on the prepared baking sheet.

5. Bake for 15•20 minutes, until the mushrooms are tender and the filling is lightly browned.

Nutritional Information:

• Calories: Approximately 50•75 calories per stuffed mushroom

• This dish would not be considered 0 points for weight loss, as the combination of the quinoa, Parmesan cheese, and breadcrumbs contributes a moderate amount of calories and macronutrients.

While the quinoa and mushrooms provide nutritional benefits, the overall calorie and macronutrient content of the stuffed mushrooms would need to be considered in a weight loss plan. The portion size and frequency of consumption would need to be carefully monitored to fit within your daily calorie and macronutrient goals.

81. Baked cinnamon apples

Ingredients:

- 4 medium apples, cored and sliced
- 2 tbsp brown sugar
- 1 tsp ground cinnamon
- 1/4 tsp ground nutmeg
- 1 tbsp unsalted butter, melted

Instructions:

1. Preheat the oven to 375°F. Grease a baking dish.

2. Arrange the apple slices in the prepared baking dish.

3. In a small bowl, mix together the brown sugar, cinnamon, and nutmeg. Sprinkle the mixture evenly over the apple slices.

4. Drizzle the melted butter over the top.

5. Bake for 20•25 minutes, until the apples are tender and the topping is lightly browned.

6. Serve warm, optionally with a scoop of vanilla ice cream or whipped cream.

Nutritional Information:

- Calories: Approximately 150•200 calories per serving

- This dish would not be considered 0 points for weight loss, as the combination of the apples, brown sugar, and butter contributes a moderate amount of calories and natural sugars.

While apples are a healthy, low•calorie fruit, the addition of the brown sugar and butter in this recipe increases the overall calorie and carbohydrate content. For a weight loss plan, the portion size and frequency of consumption would need to be carefully monitored to fit within your daily calorie and macronutrient goals.

82. Green pea soup

Ingredients:

- 2 cups frozen green peas
- 1 cup low•sodium vegetable or chicken broth
- 1/2 cup unsweetened almond milk
- 1 tbsp olive oil
- 1 shallot, diced
- 2 cloves garlic, minced
- 1 tsp fresh thyme leaves
- Salt and pepper to taste
- Chopped fresh parsley for garnish (optional)

Instructions:

1. In a saucepan, heat the olive oil over medium heat. Add the diced shallot and minced garlic. Cook for 2•3 minutes until fragrant.

2. Add the frozen green peas, vegetable or chicken broth, and thyme. Bring to a simmer and cook for 5•7 minutes, until the peas are tender.

3. Remove from heat and use an immersion blender to puree the soup until smooth. Alternatively, transfer the soup to a blender and blend until smooth.

4. Stir in the unsweetened almond milk and season with salt and pepper to taste.

5. Serve the green pea soup warm, garnished with chopped fresh parsley if desired.

Nutritional Information:

- Calories: Approximately 150•200 calories per serving

- This dish would not be considered 0 points for weight loss, as the combination of the peas, broth, and almond milk contributes a moderate amount of calories and carbohydrates.

While the green peas and other ingredients provide nutritional benefits, the overall calorie and carbohydrate content of the soup would need to be considered in a weight loss plan. The portion size and frequency of consumption would need to be carefully monitored to fit within your daily calorie and macronutrient goals.

83. Cauliflower tabbouleh

Ingredients:

- 1 head of cauliflower, florets only
- 1/2 cup chopped fresh parsley
- 1/4 cup chopped fresh mint
- 1/4 cup chopped green onions
- 2 tbsp lemon juice
- 2 tbsp olive oil
- 1 tsp ground cumin
- 1/4 tsp salt
- 1/4 tsp black pepper

Instructions:

1. In a food processor, pulse the cauliflower florets until they resemble the texture of cooked bulgur wheat.

2. Transfer the riced cauliflower to a large bowl and add the chopped parsley, mint, and green onions.

3. In a small bowl, whisk together the lemon juice, olive oil, cumin, salt, and pepper.

4. Pour the dressing over the cauliflower tabbouleh and toss to combine.

5. Chill the tabbouleh in the refrigerator for at least 30 minutes before serving.

Nutritional Information:

- Calories: Approximately 150•200 calories per serving

- This dish would not be considered 0 points for weight loss, as the combination of the cauliflower, olive oil, and herbs contributes a moderate amount of calories and fat.

While the cauliflower is a low•calorie, nutrient•dense vegetable, the addition of the olive oil and herbs increases the overall calorie and fat content of the tabbouleh. For a weight loss plan, the portion size and frequency of consumption would need to be carefully monitored to fit within your daily calorie and macronutrient goals.

84. Grilled tuna steaks with salsa verde

Ingredients:

Tuna Steaks:
• 4 (6 oz) tuna steaks
• 1 tbsp olive oil
• Salt and pepper to taste

Salsa Verde:
• 1/2 cup chopped fresh parsley
• 2 tbsp chopped fresh basil
• 2 tbsp chopped fresh oregano
• 2 tbsp capers, rinsed and chopped
• 2 tbsp lemon juice
• 1 clove garlic, minced
• 2 tbsp olive oil
• Salt and pepper to taste

Instructions:
1. Prepare the salsa verde by combining all the ingredients in a small bowl. Set aside.

2. Preheat grill or grill pan to medium•high heat.

3. Brush the tuna steaks with 1 tbsp of olive oil and season with salt and pepper.

4. Grill the tuna steaks for 2•3 minutes per side, or until cooked to your desired doneness.

5. Serve the grilled tuna steaks topped with the salsa verde.

Nutritional Information:
• Calories: Approximately 250•300 calories per serving

• This dish would not be considered 0 points for weight loss, as the combination of the tuna, olive oil, and salsa verde contributes a moderate amount of calories and fat.

While tuna is a lean protein and the salsa verde provides healthy fats and herbs, the overall calorie and macronutrient content of the dish would need to be considered in a weight loss plan. The portion size and frequency of consumption would need to be carefully monitored to fit within your daily calorie and macronutrient goals.

85. Asian slaw with sesame ginger dressing

Ingredients:

Slaw:
- 2 cups shredded green cabbage
- 1 cup shredded red cabbage
- 1 cup shredded carrots
- 1/2 cup thinly sliced snow peas
- 2 tbsp chopped fresh cilantro

Dressing:
- 2 tbsp rice vinegar
- 1 tbsp sesame oil
- 1 tbsp grated fresh ginger
- 1 tsp honey
- 1 tsp Dijon mustard
- 1 clove garlic, minced
- 1/4 tsp salt
- 1/4 tsp black pepper

Instructions:

1. In a large bowl, combine the shredded green cabbage, red cabbage, carrots, snow peas, and cilantro.

2. In a small bowl, whisk together all the dressing ingredients.

3. Pour the dressing over the slaw and toss to coat evenly.

4. Chill the Asian slaw in the refrigerator for at least 30 minutes before serving.

Nutritional Information:
- Calories: Approximately 150•200 calories per serving

- This dish would not be considered 0 points for weight loss, as the combination of the vegetables, sesame oil, and other dressing ingredients contributes a moderate amount of calories and fat.

While the slaw is made up of nutrient•dense vegetables, the addition of the sesame oil and other dressing components increases the overall calorie and fat content. For a weight loss plan, the portion size and frequency of consumption would need to be carefully monitored to fit within your daily calorie and macronutrient goals.

86. Stuffed zucchini boats

Ingredients:

• 4 medium zucchini, halved lengthwise
• 1 lb ground turkey or lean ground beef
• 1/2 cup diced onion
• 2 cloves garlic, minced
• 1 cup marinara sauce
• 1/2 cup shredded mozzarella cheese
• 2 tbsp grated Parmesan cheese
• 1 tsp dried oregano
• Salt and pepper to taste

Instructions:

1. Preheat the oven to 375°F. Scoop out the flesh from the zucchini halves, leaving a 1/4•inch shell. Finely chop the zucchini flesh.

2. In a skillet, cook the ground turkey or beef over medium heat until browned and crumbled. Drain any excess fat.

3. Add the diced onion and minced garlic to the skillet. Cook for 2•3 minutes until fragrant.

4. Stir in the chopped zucchini flesh, marinara sauce, 1/4 cup of the mozzarella cheese, Parmesan cheese, and oregano. Season with salt and pepper.

5. Spoon the filling into the zucchini boats and place them in a baking dish.

6. Top the stuffed zucchini boats with the remaining 1/4 cup mozzarella cheese.

7. Bake for 20•25 minutes, until the zucchini is tender and the cheese is melted.

Nutritional Information:
• Calories: Approximately 250•300 calories per stuffed zucchini boat
• This dish would not be considered 0 points for weight loss, as the combination of the ground meat, cheese, and marinara sauce contributes a significant amount of calories and macronutrients.

While the zucchini provides a low•calorie base, the overall calorie and macronutrient content of the stuffed zucchini boats would need to be considered in a weight loss plan. The portion size and frequency of consumption would need to be carefully monitored to fit within your daily calorie and macronutrient goals.

87. Cabbage and carrot salad with lemon vinaigrette

Ingredients:

Salad:
• 4 cups shredded green cabbage
• 2 cups shredded carrots
• 1/4 cup chopped fresh parsley

Vinaigrette:
• 2 tbsp lemon juice
• 1 tbsp olive oil
• 1 tsp Dijon mustard
• 1 tsp honey
• 1/4 tsp salt
• 1/4 tsp black pepper

Instructions:

1. In a large bowl, combine the shredded green cabbage, carrots, and chopped parsley.

2. In a small bowl, whisk together the lemon juice, olive oil, Dijon mustard, honey, salt, and pepper to make the vinaigrette.

3. Pour the vinaigrette over the cabbage and carrot salad and toss to coat evenly.

4. Chill the salad in the refrigerator for at least 30 minutes before serving.

Nutritional Information:
• Calories: Approximately 150•200 calories per serving

• This dish would not be considered 0 points for weight loss, as the combination of the vegetables and the vinaigrette contributes a moderate amount of calories and fat.

While the cabbage and carrots are low•calorie, nutrient•dense vegetables, the addition of the olive oil•based vinaigrette increases the overall calorie and fat content of the salad. For a weight loss plan, the portion size and frequency of consumption would need to be carefully monitored to fit within your daily calorie and macronutrient goals.

88. Roasted pumpkin seeds

Ingredients:

• 1 cup raw pumpkin seeds (pepitas)
• 1 tbsp olive oil
• 1 tsp salt (or to taste)
• 1/2 tsp ground cumin (optional)
• 1/2 tsp chili powder (optional)

Instructions:

1. Preheat the oven to 325°F.

2. Toss the raw pumpkin seeds with the olive oil, salt, and any optional seasonings (cumin, chili powder) in a bowl.

3. Spread the seasoned pumpkin seeds in a single layer on a baking sheet.

4. Roast for 15•20 minutes, stirring occasionally, until the seeds are lightly golden and crispy.

5. Allow the roasted pumpkin seeds to cool completely before serving.

Nutritional Information:
• Calories: Approximately 150•200 calories per 1/4 cup serving

• This dish would not be considered 0 points for weight loss, as the pumpkin seeds contain a significant amount of calories and fat.

While pumpkin seeds are a nutritious snack, they are relatively high in calories and fat compared to other low•calorie options. The portion size and frequency of consumption would need to be carefully monitored in a weight loss plan to fit within your daily calorie and macronutrient goals.

89. Turkey and vegetable stir•fry

Ingredients:

- 1 lb ground turkey
- 2 tbsp sesame oil
- 2 cups mixed vegetables (e.g., broccoli, bell peppers, snow peas, carrots)
- 2 cloves garlic, minced
- 1 tbsp grated fresh ginger
- 2 tbsp low•sodium soy sauce
- 1 tbsp rice vinegar
- 1 tsp honey
- Salt and pepper to taste
- Cooked brown rice, for serving

Instructions:

1. In a large skillet or wok, cook the ground turkey over medium•high heat, breaking it up as it cooks, until browned and cooked through, about 5•7 minutes. Transfer the turkey to a plate.

2. Add the sesame oil to the skillet. Add the mixed vegetables, garlic, and ginger. Stir•fry for 5•7 minutes, until the vegetables are tender•crisp.

3. Return the cooked turkey to the skillet. Add the soy sauce, rice vinegar, and honey. Toss to combine and heat through.

4. Season with salt and pepper to taste.

5. Serve the turkey and vegetable stir•fry over cooked brown rice.

Nutritional Information:
- Calories: Approximately 300•400 calories per serving (with 1/2 cup brown rice)
- This dish would not be considered 0 points for weight loss, as the combination of the turkey, vegetables, and stir•fry sauce contributes a moderate amount of calories and macronutrients.

While the turkey and vegetables provide nutritional benefits, the overall calorie and macronutrient content of the stir•fry would need to be considered in a weight loss plan. The portion size and frequency of consumption would need to be carefully monitored to fit within your daily calorie and macronutrient goals.

90. Mixed berry salad with mint

Ingredients:

- 1 cup fresh strawberries, halved
- 1 cup fresh blueberries
- 1 cup fresh raspberries
- 1/4 cup fresh mint leaves, chopped
- 1 tbsp honey
- 1 tbsp lemon juice

Instructions:

1. In a large bowl, gently combine the halved strawberries, blueberries, raspberries, and chopped mint leaves.

2. In a small bowl, whisk together the honey and lemon juice to make a simple dressing.

3. Drizzle the honey•lemon dressing over the mixed berries and mint. Toss gently to coat.

4. Serve the mixed berry salad chilled or at room temperature.

Nutritional Information:

- Calories: Approximately 150•200 calories per serving

- This dish would not be considered 0 points for weight loss, as the combination of the berries and honey dressing contributes a moderate amount of natural sugars and calories.

While the berries and mint provide nutritional benefits, the addition of the honey in the dressing increases the overall calorie and carbohydrate content of the salad. For a weight loss plan, the portion size and frequency of consumption would need to be carefully monitored to fit within your daily calorie and macronutrient goals.

91. Ratatouille stuffed bell peppers

Ingredients:

- 4 bell peppers, halved and seeded
- 1 tbsp olive oil
- 1 onion, diced
- 2 cloves garlic, minced
- 1 eggplant, diced
- 1 zucchini, diced
- 1 can (14 oz) diced tomatoes
- 2 tbsp tomato paste
- 1 tsp dried oregano
- 1/4 tsp red pepper flakes (optional)
- Salt and pepper to taste
- 1/2 cup shredded mozzarella cheese

Instructions:

1. Preheat the oven to 375°F. Place the bell pepper halves in a baking dish.

2. In a skillet, heat the olive oil over medium heat. Add the onion and garlic, and sauté for 2·3 minutes.

3. Add the diced eggplant and zucchini to the skillet. Cook for 5·7 minutes, until the vegetables are tender.

4. Stir in the diced tomatoes, tomato paste, oregano, and red pepper flakes (if using). Season with salt and pepper. Spoon the ratatouille mixture into the bell pepper halves, packing it in gently.

5. Top the stuffed peppers with the shredded mozzarella cheese. Bake for 20·25 minutes, until the peppers are tender and the cheese is melted.

Nutritional Information:
- Calories: Approximately 250·300 calories per stuffed pepper
- This dish would not be considered 0 points for weight loss, as the combination of the vegetables, tomato sauce, and cheese contributes a moderate amount of calories and macronutrients.

While the bell peppers, eggplant, and zucchini provide nutritional benefits, the overall calorie and macronutrient content of the stuffed peppers would need to be considered in a weight loss plan. The portion size and frequency of consumption would need to be carefully monitored to fit within your daily calorie and macronutrient goals.

92. Baked cod with lemon and capers

Ingredients:

- 1 lb cod fillets
- 2 tbsp olive oil
- 2 tbsp lemon juice
- 2 tbsp capers, rinsed and chopped
- 2 cloves garlic, minced
- 1 tsp dried parsley
- Salt and pepper to taste

Instructions:

1. Preheat the oven to 400°F. Grease a baking dish.

2. Place the cod fillets in the prepared baking dish.

3. In a small bowl, whisk together the olive oil, lemon juice, capers, garlic, and dried parsley.

4. Pour the lemon•caper mixture over the cod fillets, making sure to evenly coat them.

5. Season the cod with salt and pepper.

6. Bake for 15•20 minutes, or until the cod is opaque and flakes easily with a fork.

7. Serve the baked cod immediately, garnished with additional lemon wedges if desired.

Nutritional Information:

- Calories: Approximately 200•250 calories per serving

- This dish would not be considered 0 points for weight loss, as the combination of the cod, olive oil, and capers contributes a moderate amount of calories and fat.

While cod is a lean, protein•rich fish, the addition of the olive oil and capers increases the overall calorie and fat content of the dish. For a weight loss plan, the portion size and frequency of consumption would need to be carefully monitored to fit within your daily calorie and macronutrient goals.

93. Spinach and lentil salad

Ingredients:

- 4 cups baby spinach
- 1 cup cooked lentils, cooled
- 1/2 cup diced cucumber
- 1/4 cup diced red onion
- 2 tbsp crumbled feta cheese
- 2 tbsp olive oil
- 1 tbsp balsamic vinegar
- 1 tsp Dijon mustard
- 1 tsp honey
- Salt and pepper to taste

Instructions:

1. In a large bowl, combine the baby spinach, cooked lentils, diced cucumber, and diced red onion.

2. In a small bowl, whisk together the olive oil, balsamic vinegar, Dijon mustard, and honey. Season with salt and pepper.

3. Drizzle the dressing over the spinach and lentil salad and toss gently to coat.

4. Top the salad with the crumbled feta cheese.

5. Serve the spinach and lentil salad chilled or at room temperature.

Nutritional Information:

- Calories: Approximately 200•250 calories per serving

- This dish would not be considered 0 points for weight loss, as the combination of the lentils, olive oil, and feta cheese contributes a moderate amount of calories and macronutrients.

While the spinach and lentils provide nutritional benefits, the addition of the olive oil•based dressing and feta cheese increases the overall calorie and fat content of the salad. For a weight loss plan, the portion size and frequency of consumption would need to be carefully monitored to fit within your daily calorie and macronutrient goals.

94. Grilled shrimp with mango salsa

Ingredients:

Shrimp:
• 1 lb large shrimp, peeled and deveined
• 1 tbsp olive oil
• 1 tsp chili powder
• 1/2 tsp garlic powder
• Salt and pepper to taste

Mango Salsa:
• 1 ripe mango, diced
• 1/2 cup diced red onion
• 1/4 cup chopped fresh cilantro
• 1 jalapeño, seeded and minced (optional)
• 2 tbsp lime juice
• 1 tbsp olive oil
• Salt and pepper to taste

Instructions:

1. In a bowl, toss the shrimp with the olive oil, chili powder, garlic powder, salt, and pepper.
2. Preheat a grill or grill pan to medium•high heat.

3. Grill the shrimp for 2•3 minutes per side, until they are opaque and cooked through.

4. In a separate bowl, combine all the mango salsa ingredients and mix well.

5. Serve the grilled shrimp topped with the mango salsa.

Nutritional Information:

• Calories: Approximately 250•300 calories per serving

• This dish would not be considered 0 points for weight loss, as the combination of the shrimp, olive oil, and mango salsa contributes a moderate amount of calories and fat.

While the shrimp and mango provide nutritional benefits, the overall calorie and macronutrient content of the dish would need to be considered in a weight loss plan. The portion size and frequency of consumption would need to be carefully monitored to fit within your daily calorie and macronutrient goals.

95. Caprese•stuffed avocado

Ingredients:

• 2 ripe avocados, halved and pitted
• 1 cup cherry tomatoes, halved
• 1/2 cup fresh mozzarella cheese, diced
• 2 tbsp fresh basil, chopped
• 1 tbsp balsamic glaze
• Salt and pepper to taste

Instructions:

1. Scoop out a small portion of the avocado flesh from the center of each avocado half, leaving a 1/2•inch border.

2. In a bowl, gently mix together the scooped•out avocado flesh, cherry tomatoes, mozzarella cheese, and fresh basil.

3. Spoon the caprese mixture back into the avocado halves.

4. Drizzle the balsamic glaze over the top of the stuffed avocados.

5. Season with salt and pepper to taste.

6. Serve the caprese•stuffed avocados immediately.

Nutritional Information:

• Calories: Approximately 250•300 calories per stuffed avocado half

• This dish would not be considered 0 points for weight loss, as the combination of the avocado, mozzarella cheese, and balsamic glaze contributes a significant amount of calories and fat.

While the avocado, tomatoes, and basil provide nutritional benefits, the overall calorie and macronutrient content of the stuffed avocado would need to be considered in a weight loss plan. The portion size and frequency of consumption would need to be carefully monitored to fit within your daily calorie and macronutrient goals.

96. Greek yogurt with mixed nuts

Ingredients:

• 1 cup plain Greek yogurt
• 2 tablespoons mixed nuts (such as almonds, walnuts, pecans)
• 1 teaspoon honey (optional)

Instructions:

1. Scoop the Greek yogurt into a bowl.

2. Sprinkle the mixed nuts on top of the yogurt.

3. If desired, drizzle the honey over the top.

Nutrition Information (per serving):
• Calories: 200
• Total Fat: 12g
• Saturated Fat: 2g
• Carbohydrates: 10g
• Fiber: 3g
• Protein: 15g

This recipe is a great source of protein, healthy fats, and fiber. The Greek yogurt provides probiotics, while the nuts add crunch and additional nutrients. This makes for a satisfying and nutritious snack or light meal.

In terms of weight loss, this recipe is considered 0 points as it is a relatively low•calorie, high•protein option that can be part of a balanced diet. The healthy fats and fiber from the nuts also help promote feelings of fullness.

97. Cucumber noodle salad with peanut dressing

Ingredients:

• 2 medium cucumbers, spiralized or julienned into noodles
• 1/2 cup shredded carrots
• 1/4 cup chopped fresh cilantro
• 2 tablespoons chopped roasted peanuts

For the Peanut Dressing:
• 2 tablespoons creamy peanut butter
• 2 tablespoons rice vinegar
• 1 tablespoon low•sodium soy sauce
• 1 teaspoon sesame oil
• 1 teaspoon honey
• 1 teaspoon grated fresh ginger
• 1•2 tablespoons water to thin the dressing

Instructions:

1. In a large bowl, combine the cucumber noodles, carrots, cilantro, and peanuts.

2. In a small bowl, whisk together all the dressing ingredients until smooth. Add water as needed to reach desired consistency.

3. Pour the peanut dressing over the salad and toss to coat evenly.

4. Serve chilled or at room temperature.

Nutrition Information (per serving):
• Calories: 120
• Total Fat: 7g
• Saturated Fat: 1g
• Carbohydrates: 12g
• Fiber: 3g
• Protein: 4g

This cucumber noodle salad is a refreshing and flavorful dish that is low in calories and high in nutrients. The peanut dressing adds a creamy, nutty flavor that complements the crunchy vegetables. This recipe is considered 0 points for weight loss as it is a low•calorie, high•fiber option that can be enjoyed as a light meal or side dish.

98. Stuffed cherry tomatoes with tuna

Ingredients:

- 12 cherry tomatoes
- 1 (5 oz) can tuna, drained
- 2 tablespoons plain Greek yogurt
- 1 tablespoon finely chopped fresh parsley
- 1 teaspoon lemon juice
- Salt and pepper to taste

Instructions:

1. Slice the top off each cherry tomato and scoop out the seeds and pulp, leaving a small hollow shell.

2. In a small bowl, mix together the tuna, Greek yogurt, parsley, and lemon juice. Season with salt and pepper.

3. Spoon the tuna mixture into the hollowed·out tomato shells.

4. Arrange the stuffed tomatoes on a serving plate and chill in the refrigerator until ready to serve.

Nutrition Information (per serving, 2 stuffed tomatoes):
- Calories: 50
- Total Fat: 1g
- Saturated Fat: 0g
- Carbohydrates: 3g
- Fiber: 1g
- Protein: 7g

This recipe for Stuffed Cherry Tomatoes with Tuna is a great low·calorie, high·protein option that is perfect for weight loss. The tuna provides a good source of lean protein, while the cherry tomatoes are low in calories and high in vitamins and antioxidants. This dish is considered 0 points for weight loss as it is a nutrient·dense, low·calorie snack or appetizer that can be enjoyed as part of a balanced diet.

99. Steamed artichokes with lemon garlic aioli

Ingredients:

For the Artichokes:
• 2 medium artichokes
• 1 lemon, cut in half
• 1 cup water

For the Lemon Garlic Aioli:
• 1/2 cup mayonnaise
• 2 cloves garlic, minced
• 1 tablespoon lemon juice
• 1 teaspoon Dijon mustard
• Salt and pepper to taste

Instructions:

1. Prepare the artichokes:
   • Trim the stem of each artichoke, leaving about 1 inch. Snip off the thorny tips of the leaves using kitchen shears.
   • Place the artichokes in a steamer basket and add the water. Squeeze the lemon halves over the artichokes and add the squeezed lemon halves to the steamer.
   • Steam the artichokes for 25•30 minutes, or until the leaves pull off easily.

2. Make the Lemon Garlic Aioli:
   • In a small bowl, whisk together the mayonnaise, garlic, lemon juice, and Dijon mustard. Season with salt and pepper to taste.

3. Serve the steamed artichokes warm, with the lemon garlic aioli on the side for dipping.

Nutrition Information (per serving, 1/2 artichoke with 2 tbsp aioli):
• Calories: 120
• Total Fat: 9g
• Saturated Fat: 1.5g
• Carbohydrates: 8g
• Fiber: 4g
• Protein: 3g

This recipe for Steamed Artichokes with Lemon Garlic Aioli is a great low•calorie, low•carb option that is perfect for weight loss. The artichokes are a good source of fiber and antioxidants, while the aioli provides a flavorful dipping sauce without adding too many calories. This dish is considered 0 points for weight loss as it is a nutrient•dense, low•calorie option that can be enjoyed as part of a balanced diet.

100. Broccoli and cauliflower gratin

Ingredients:

• 1 head broccoli, cut into florets
• 1 head cauliflower, cut into florets
• 2 tablespoons olive oil
• 2 cloves garlic, minced
• 2 tablespoons all•purpose flour
• 1 cup low•fat milk
• 1/2 cup low•sodium chicken or vegetable broth
• 1/2 cup shredded low•fat cheddar cheese
• 1/4 cup grated Parmesan cheese
• Salt and pepper to taste
• 2 tablespoons panko breadcrumbs

Instructions:

1. Preheat the oven to 375°F.

2. In a large pot, bring a few inches of water to a boil. Add the broccoli and cauliflower florets and steam for 5•7 minutes, until tender•crisp. Drain and set aside.

3. In a saucepan, heat the olive oil over medium heat. Add the garlic and cook for 1 minute, until fragrant.

4. Whisk in the flour and cook for 1 minute. Gradually whisk in the milk and broth, and cook until the sauce thickens, about 5 minutes.

5. Remove the sauce from heat and stir in the cheddar and Parmesan cheeses. Season with salt and pepper.

6. Arrange the steamed broccoli and cauliflower in a baking dish. Pour the cheese sauce over the top and sprinkle with the panko breadcrumbs.

7. Bake for 20•25 minutes, until the top is golden brown and bubbly.

This Broccoli and Cauliflower Gratin is a delicious and nutritious side dish that is perfect for weight loss. The vegetables provide fiber and essential vitamins and minerals, while the cheese sauce adds a creamy, satisfying element without too many calories. This dish is considered 0 points for weight loss as it is a low•calorie, nutrient•dense option that can be enjoyed as part of a balanced diet.

101. Turkey and bean chili

Ingredients:

- 1 lb ground turkey
- 1 onion, diced
- 3 cloves garlic, minced
- 2 tablespoons chili powder
- 1 teaspoon cumin
- 1 teaspoon oregano
- 1/2 teaspoon smoked paprika
- 1/4 teaspoon cayenne pepper (optional)
- 1 (15 oz) can diced tomatoes
- 1 (15 oz) can kidney beans, rinsed and drained
- 1 (15 oz) can black beans, rinsed and drained
- 1 cup low•sodium chicken or vegetable broth
- Salt and pepper to taste
- Chopped fresh cilantro for serving (optional)

Instructions:

1. In a large pot or Dutch oven, cook the ground turkey over medium•high heat, breaking it up with a wooden spoon, until browned and cooked through, about 5•7 minutes.

2. Add the onion and garlic and cook for 2•3 minutes until softened.

3. Stir in the chili powder, cumin, oregano, smoked paprika, and cayenne (if using). Cook for 1 minute to toast the spices.

4. Add the diced tomatoes, kidney beans, black beans, and broth. Bring to a simmer and let cook for 15•20 minutes, stirring occasionally, until the flavors have melded and the chili has thickened.

5. Season with salt and pepper to taste. Serve the chili hot, garnished with chopped fresh cilantro if desired.

Nutrition Information (per serving, 1 cup):
- Calories: 250
- Total Fat: 5g
- Saturated Fat: 1g
- Carbohydrates: 30g
- Fiber: 10g
- Protein: 25g

102. Bell pepper nachos with ground turkey

Ingredients:

• 2 large bell peppers, sliced into 1/2•inch thick rounds
• 1 lb ground turkey
• 1 tablespoon olive oil
• 1 onion, diced
• 2 cloves garlic, minced
• 1 tablespoon chili powder
• 1 teaspoon cumin
• 1/2 teaspoon oregano
• Salt and pepper to taste
• 1/2 cup shredded low•fat cheddar cheese
• 2 tablespoons chopped fresh cilantro (optional)

Instructions:

1. Preheat the oven to 400°F.

2. Arrange the bell pepper slices in a single layer on a baking sheet. Bake for 10•12 minutes, until slightly softened.

3. In a large skillet, cook the ground turkey over medium•high heat, breaking it up with a wooden spoon, until browned and cooked through, about 5•7 minutes.

4. Add the olive oil, onion, and garlic to the skillet. Cook for 2•3 minutes until the onion is translucent.

5. Stir in the chili powder, cumin, oregano, and a pinch of salt and pepper. Cook for 1 minute to toast the spices.

6. Remove the bell pepper slices from the oven and top with the seasoned ground turkey mixture.

7. Sprinkle the shredded cheddar cheese over the top.

8. Return the nachos to the oven and bake for 5•7 minutes, until the cheese is melted and bubbly. Garnish with chopped fresh cilantro, if desired.

These Bell Pepper Nachos with Ground Turkey are a delicious and healthy alternative to traditional nachos. The bell pepper slices act as the "chips," while the lean ground turkey and low•fat cheese provide a satisfying and protein•rich topping. This recipe is considered 0 points for weight loss as it is a low•calorie, nutrient•dense option that can be enjoyed as part of a balanced diet.

103. Strawberry spinach salad with poppyseed dressing

Ingredients:

For the Salad:
• 5 oz baby spinach
• 1 cup fresh strawberries, sliced
• 1/4 cup sliced almonds
• 2 tablespoons crumbled feta cheese (optional)

For the Poppy Seed Dressing:
• 2 tablespoons white wine vinegar
• 1 tablespoon honey
• 1 tablespoon Dijon mustard
• 1 tablespoon poppy seeds
• 2 tablespoons olive oil
• Salt and pepper to taste

Instructions:

1. In a large salad bowl, combine the baby spinach, sliced strawberries, sliced almonds, and crumbled feta cheese (if using).

2. In a small bowl, whisk together the white wine vinegar, honey, Dijon mustard, and poppy seeds. Slowly drizzle in the olive oil while whisking constantly until the dressing is emulsified. Season with salt and pepper to taste.

3. Just before serving, drizzle the poppy seed dressing over the salad and toss gently to coat.

Nutrition Information (per serving, 1/4 of the salad):
• Calories: 150
• Total Fat: 10g
• Saturated Fat: 2g
• Carbohydrates: 12g
• Fiber: 3g
• Protein: 4g

This Strawberry Spinach Salad with Poppy Seed Dressing is a delicious and nutritious option that is perfect for weight loss. The spinach and strawberries provide a good source of fiber, vitamins, and antioxidants, while the poppy seed dressing adds a flavorful and creamy element without too many calories. This recipe is considered 0 points for weight loss as it is a low•calorie, nutrient•dense option that can be enjoyed as part of a balanced diet.

104. Seared tuna salad with ginger dressing

Ingredients:

For the Salad:
• 8 oz sushi•grade tuna steak
• 1 tablespoon olive oil
• 5 oz mixed greens
• 1/2 cup sliced cucumber
• 1/4 cup shredded carrots
• 2 tablespoons toasted sesame seeds

For the Ginger Dressing:
• 2 tablespoons rice vinegar
• 1 tablespoon low•sodium soy sauce
• 1 tablespoon honey
• 1 teaspoon grated fresh ginger
• 1 teaspoon sesame oil
• 1 tablespoon olive oil
• Salt and pepper to taste

Instructions:

1. In a small bowl, whisk together all the dressing ingredients until well combined. Set aside.

2. Heat a large skillet over high heat. Rub the tuna steak with the olive oil and season with salt and pepper.

3. Sear the tuna for 1•2 minutes per side, or until the outside is lightly browned but the center is still rare. Remove from heat and let rest for 5 minutes, then slice into thin strips.

4. In a large salad bowl, combine the mixed greens, cucumber, carrots, and toasted sesame seeds.

5. Drizzle the ginger dressing over the salad and toss to coat. Top the salad with the seared tuna slices and serve immediately.

Nutrition Information (per serving, 1/2 of the salad):
• Calories: 300
• Total Fat: 16g
• Saturated Fat: 2g
• Carbohydrates: 14g
• Fiber: 3g
• Protein: 27g

105. Garlic roasted broccoli

Ingredients:

- 1 lb broccoli florets
- 2 tablespoons olive oil
- 3 cloves garlic, minced
- 1/4 teaspoon red pepper flakes (optional)
- Salt and pepper to taste
- 1 tablespoon lemon juice (optional)

Instructions:

1. Preheat the oven to 400°F.

2. In a large bowl, toss the broccoli florets with the olive oil, garlic, red pepper flakes (if using), and a pinch of salt and pepper.

3. Spread the broccoli in a single layer on a baking sheet.

4. Roast for 15•20 minutes, tossing halfway, until the broccoli is tender and lightly browned.

5. Remove the broccoli from the oven and drizzle with the lemon juice, if using. Toss to coat. Serve hot.

Nutrition Information (per serving, about 1 cup):
- Calories: 80
- Total Fat: 5g
- Saturated Fat: 1g
- Carbohydrates: 7g
- Fiber: 3g
- Protein: 3g

This Garlic Roasted Broccoli is a simple and delicious side dish that is perfect for weight loss. Broccoli is a nutrient•dense vegetable that is low in calories and high in fiber, vitamins, and antioxidants. The garlic and optional red pepper flakes add flavor without adding too many calories. This recipe is considered 0 points for weight loss as it is a low•calorie, nutrient•dense option that can be enjoyed as part of a balanced diet.

106. Turkey sausage with peppers and onions

Ingredients:

- 1 lb turkey sausage links, sliced into 1/2·inch pieces
- 1 tablespoon olive oil
- 1 large bell pepper, sliced
- 1 onion, sliced
- 2 cloves garlic, minced
- 1 teaspoon dried oregano
- 1/4 teaspoon red pepper flakes (optional)
- Salt and pepper to taste

Instructions:

1. In a large skillet, heat the olive oil over medium·high heat.

2. Add the sliced turkey sausage and cook, stirring occasionally, until lightly browned, about 5·7 minutes.

3. Add the sliced bell pepper and onion to the skillet. Cook for 5·7 minutes, stirring occasionally, until the vegetables are tender.

4. Stir in the minced garlic, oregano, and red pepper flakes (if using). Cook for 1 minute until fragrant.

5. Season the mixture with salt and pepper to taste. Serve the turkey sausage and vegetable mixture hot.

Nutrition Information (per serving, about 1 cup):
- Calories: 200
- Total Fat: 10g
- Saturated Fat: 2g
- Carbohydrates: 10g
- Fiber: 3g
- Protein: 20g

This Turkey Sausage with Peppers and Onions is a delicious and nutritious dish that is perfect for weight loss. The turkey sausage provides a good source of lean protein, while the peppers and onions add fiber, vitamins, and antioxidants. This recipe is considered 0 points for weight loss as it is a low·calorie, nutrient·dense option that can be enjoyed as part of a balanced diet.

107. Greek yogurt with fresh fruit compote

Ingredients:

For the Fruit Compote:
• 2 cups mixed fresh berries (such as strawberries, blueberries, raspberries)
• 1 tablespoon honey
• 1 tablespoon water
• 1 teaspoon lemon juice

For the Yogurt:
• 1 cup plain Greek yogurt
• 1 teaspoon vanilla extract (optional)

Instructions:

1. Make the Fruit Compote:
   • In a small saucepan, combine the mixed berries, honey, water, and lemon juice.
   • Bring the mixture to a simmer over medium heat, stirring occasionally, until the berries have released their juices and the compote has thickened slightly, about 5•7 minutes.
   • Remove from heat and let cool slightly.

2. Assemble the Yogurt:
   • In a serving bowl, place the plain Greek yogurt.
   • Top the yogurt with the warm fruit compote.
   • If desired, stir in the vanilla extract.

Nutrition Information (per serving, 1/2 cup yogurt with 1/4 cup compote):
• Calories: 150
• Total Fat: 3g
• Saturated Fat: 1g
• Carbohydrates: 20g
• Fiber: 3g
• Protein: 12g

This Greek Yogurt with Fresh Fruit Compote is a delicious and nutritious breakfast or snack option that is perfect for weight loss. The Greek yogurt provides a good source of protein, while the fresh fruit compote adds natural sweetness and fiber without too many calories. This recipe is considered 0 points for weight loss as it is a low•calorie, nutrient•dense option that can be enjoyed as part of a balanced diet.

108. Asian cucumber salad

Ingredients:

• 2 medium cucumbers, thinly sliced
• 1/4 cup rice vinegar
• 1 tablespoon sesame oil
• 1 tablespoon low•sodium soy sauce
• 1 teaspoon honey
• 1 teaspoon toasted sesame seeds
• 1 tablespoon chopped fresh cilantro (optional)
• Salt and pepper to taste

Instructions:

1. In a large bowl, combine the thinly sliced cucumbers.

2. In a small bowl, whisk together the rice vinegar, sesame oil, soy sauce, and honey.

3. Pour the dressing over the cucumbers and toss to coat evenly.

4. Sprinkle the toasted sesame seeds and chopped cilantro (if using) over the top.

5. Season with salt and pepper to taste.

6. Cover and refrigerate for at least 30 minutes to allow the flavors to meld.

7. Serve chilled or at room temperature.

Nutrition Information (per serving, about 1 cup):
• Calories: 50
• Total Fat: 2g
• Saturated Fat: 0g
• Carbohydrates: 7g
• Fiber: 1g
• Protein: 1g

This Asian Cucumber Salad is a refreshing and flavorful side dish that is perfect for weight loss. The cucumbers are low in calories and high in water content, while the dressing adds a delicious blend of sweet, sour, and savory flavors without adding too many calories. This recipe is considered 0 points for weight loss as it is a low•calorie, nutrient•dense option that can be enjoyed as part of a balanced diet.

109. Baked chicken drumsticks with herbs

Ingredients:

• 8 chicken drumsticks (about 2 lbs)
• 2 tablespoons olive oil
• 1 teaspoon dried thyme
• 1 teaspoon dried rosemary
• 1 teaspoon garlic powder
• 1/2 teaspoon paprika
• Salt and pepper to taste
• Chopped fresh parsley for garnish (optional)

Instructions:

1. Preheat the oven to 400°F. Line a baking sheet with parchment paper or foil.

2. Pat the chicken drumsticks dry with paper towels and place them in a large bowl.

3. Drizzle the olive oil over the drumsticks and toss to coat evenly.

4. In a small bowl, mix together the thyme, rosemary, garlic powder, paprika, and a generous pinch of salt and pepper.

5. Sprinkle the seasoning mixture over the drumsticks and use your hands to rub it in and evenly coat the chicken.

6. Arrange the seasoned drumsticks on the prepared baking sheet, making sure they are not touching.

7. Bake for 35·40 minutes, flipping the drumsticks halfway through, until the chicken is cooked through and the skin is crispy. Garnish with chopped fresh parsley, if desired.

Nutrition Information (per serving, 2 drumsticks):
• Calories: 220
• Total Fat: 12g
• Saturated Fat: 3g
• Carbohydrates: 0g
• Fiber: 0g
• Protein: 26g

These Baked Chicken Drumsticks with Herbs are a delicious and healthy option for weight loss. The chicken is a lean protein source, and the herbs and spices add flavor without adding too many calories. This recipe is considered 0 points for weight loss as it is a low·calorie, nutrient·dense option that can be enjoyed as part of a balanced diet.

110. Grilled vegetable salad with balsamic glaze

Ingredients:

• 1 zucchini, sliced into 1/2•inch thick rounds
• 1 yellow squash, sliced into 1/2•inch thick rounds
• 1 red bell pepper, cut into 1•inch pieces
• 1 red onion, sliced into 1/2•inch thick rounds
• 2 tablespoons olive oil
• Salt and pepper to taste
• 4 cups mixed greens
• 2 tablespoons balsamic glaze

Instructions:

1. Preheat grill or grill pan to medium•high heat.

2. In a large bowl, toss the zucchini, yellow squash, bell pepper, and onion slices with the olive oil. Season with salt and pepper.

3. Grill the vegetables for 3•5 minutes per side, or until tender and lightly charred.

4. Remove the grilled vegetables from the grill and let cool slightly.

5. In a large salad bowl, arrange the mixed greens. Top with the grilled vegetables.

6. Drizzle the balsamic glaze over the salad and toss gently to coat. Serve immediately.

Nutrition Information (per serving, 1/4 of the salad):
• Calories: 120
• Total Fat: 6g
• Saturated Fat: 1g
• Carbohydrates: 12g
• Fiber: 3g
• Protein: 3g

This Grilled Vegetable Salad with Balsamic Glaze is a delicious and nutritious option that is perfect for weight loss. The grilled vegetables provide a good source of fiber, vitamins, and antioxidants, while the balsamic glaze adds a sweet and tangy flavor without too many calories. This recipe is considered 0 points for weight loss as it is a low•calorie, nutrient•dense option that can be enjoyed as part of a balanced diet.

Thank you for exploring the **0-Point Weight Loss Cookbook: Fresh, Flavorful, and Filling Recipes for Weight Loss Success.** We hope this collection of over 100 zero-point recipes has inspired you to embrace a healthier, more flavorful approach to weight loss.

As you've discovered, achieving your weight loss goals doesn't require deprivation or bland, uninteresting meals. By focusing on zero-point foods, you can enjoy a wide variety of delicious and satisfying dishes that nourish your body and support your journey towards a healthier you.

Moving Forward

Your journey towards weight loss success is unique, and it's important to find what works best for you. Use this cookbook as a foundation, but feel free to experiment, adapt, and personalize the recipes to suit your preferences and needs. The key is to enjoy the process and make it your own.

Remember, every small step you take towards healthier eating and living is a step in the right direction. Celebrate your progress, be kind to yourself, and stay committed to your goals. Weight loss is a journey, and with the right tools and mindset, it's a journey you can enjoy and succeed in.

Final Thoughts

We hope this cookbook has provided you with not only a wealth of delicious zero-point recipes but also the inspiration and confidence to take charge of your weight loss journey. Eating healthy doesn't have to be a struggle; it can be a delightful and rewarding experience.

Thank you for letting us be a part of your journey. Here's to your continued success, health, and happiness. May your kitchen be filled with the aromas of fresh, flavorful, and filling dishes that support your goals and bring joy to your table.

Happy cooking, and enjoy every bite!

9 798328 447393